Treating Drug Abusers

Edited by
Gerald Bennett

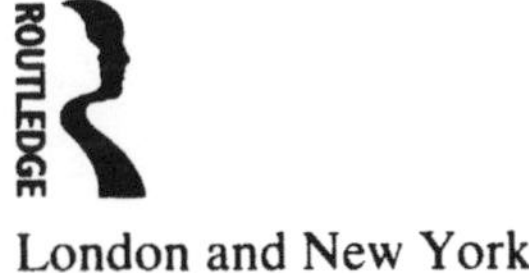

London and New York

First published 1989
by Routledge
2 Park Square, Milton Park, Abingdon, Oxon, OX14 4RN

Simultaneously published in the USA and Canada
by Routledge
270 Madison Ave, New York NY 10016

First published in paperback by
Routledge in 1990

Reprinted in 1993

Transferred to Digital Printing 2005

A Tavistock/Routledge publication

British Library Cataloguing in Publication Data

Treating Drug Abusers
1. Drug abuse. Treatment
I. Bennett, Gerald, *1951–*
362.2′938

Library of Congress Cataloging in Publication Data

Treating Drug Abusers/edited by Gerald Bennett.
p. cm.
Includes bibliographies and index.
1. Drug abuse – Treatment. 2. Narcotic addicts – mental health services. 3. Community mental health services. I. Bennett, Gerald 1951–
[DNLM: 1. Substance Abuse – prevention & control. 2. Substance Abuse – therapy. WM 270 T7817]
RC564.T73 1989
616.86′3 – dc19
DNLM/DLC
for Library of Congress 88–39217 CIP

ISBN 0–415–05837–6

Contents

Contributors

Gerald Bennett is a Clinical Psychologist with the East Dorset Community Drug Team, based in Bournemouth.

Henck van Bilsen is a Clinical Psychologist in the Netherlands, based at Rotterdam.

Nas Choudry is the Consultant Psychiatrist at St Anns Hospital, Poole, Dorset.

Sue Clement is a Clinical Psychologist at Dykebar Hospital in Paisley.

Paul Davis is a Clinical Psychologist with the ACORN Project in Surrey.

Stewart Dickson is the Director of AIDSLINK.

Andree van Emst is a Clinical Psychologist in the Netherlands, based at Woerden.

Moira Hamlin is a Clinical Psychologist and Head of the Community Centre for Addiction in Birmingham.

Diane Hammersley is a Psychologist with the Community Centre for Addiction in Birmingham, working on the WITHDRAW Project.

Jane Hollis is the Assistant Director of Alpha House, Droxford, Hampshire.

Geraldine Mulleady is a Clinical Psychologist with the Drug Dependency Centre at St Mary's Hospital, London.

Contributors

Will Nuzum is a 'Lifeline' Worker with the Rochdale Community Drug Team.

Claire Robbins is a Nurse Specialist with the Drug Dependency Centre at St Mary's Hospital, London.

Justine Schneider was formerly a Social Worker with the ACORN Project in Surrey.

Mike Scott is a Research Social Worker with the Liverpool Personal Service Society.

Gillian Tober is the Tutor in Addiction at the Leeds Addiction Unit.

Jenny Wilks is a Clinical Psychologist with the Maudsley Drug Training Unit, Camberwell, London.

Dennis Yandoli is a Social Worker with the Drug Dependency Centre at St Mary's Hospital, London.

Chapter One

Introduction

Gerald Bennett

This book has been written for those attempting to help drug users, with the practical aim of aiding them to improve their work with individuals and to develop their services. It has been written by drug workers and is based largely on what they have learned from their clinical experience, together with theory and research findings which have proved helpful. The practical aim shows itself in the detailed, often prescriptive, accounts written about therapeutic approaches; much of this work makes little reference to research findings which can validate or guide the tasks which drug services face – this is because such research has never been carried out. One of the chapters is exceptional in reporting the first findings of a scientific evaluation of one particular therapeutic approach, but for the most part practice has gone beyond research, and is guided by an amalgam of experience and theory.

Several important themes run through the contents of this book. Two of these, which are central concerns of Tober's contribution (Chapter 2), are the importance of learning, and the developing nature of motivation. Others are the roles of pharmacological treatments and the potential for new drug services to learn from elsewhere, principally alcohol agencies and drug agencies in the past.

The importance of learning

Drug users learn to use drugs through processes which are not unique to them, but are common to most areas of life; these operate in the individual in their own unique set of circumstances. In Chapter 2 Tober describes some of the ways in which learning processes can be involved when people learn to take drugs in different ways, including dependent use, and the factors involved in maintaining these habits. This perspective explains that people continue to take drugs, not because they have an illness or are totally irrational, but because this activity has short-term advantages for them which outweigh the long-term disadvantages. The potential gains that may even occur for the families of drug users are explored in the chapter on family perspectives and family therapy by Yandoli and his colleagues (Chapter 4). The importance of learning is also relevant for drug users when they wish to stop taking drugs. They may need to develop alternative means of achieving some of the benefits that drug taking brings them, or of developing skills to better cope with areas of life that are problematic and may increase their vulnerability to the attractions of drugs. Such skills might, for example, aid them to achieve independence from their parents or to cope with symptoms of anxiety. In their chapter on AIDS Dickson and Hollis argue strongly that developing attractive alternative skills is crucial where change in sexual practices is advocated. There may also be value in unlearning ingrained responses to certain situations, such as the automatic craving that may accompany handling syringes.

The process of learning is seldom error-free, and there is little reason to expect that drug users who are learning to live without drugs should be able to achieve this successfully at the first attempt. As Scott points out in his chapter on relapse prevention training (Chapter 5) drug services have not always absorbed the implications of the notion that mistakes are important learning experiences, and the fact that most people who do become lastingly drug free do so as a result of a stuttering series of unsuccessful attempts. Scott's contribution describes therapeutic approaches to facilitate this process.

The developing nature of motivation

This book represents a move away from the over-simple view of drug users as being either motivated or not-motivated to stop using drugs (with the implication that only motivated users can be helped). Most chapters refer to the stages of change model of Prochaska and DiClemente (1984) which argues that drug users who stop, go through a predictable sequence of different stages in which their motivation develops and changes. This view has had a practical implication of pointing out the differing needs of people in different stages of change, so that comprehensive services should serve each appropriately; the injecting drug user who is determined to continue taking drugs, the user who is thinking of stopping, the person who is actively trying to stop, and the person who has been stopped for some time. Dickson and Hollis (Chapter 8) describe some of the practical ways in which determined drug users can be helped to protect themselves from the potentially fatal HIV infection. If the nature of motivation can develop and change in predictable ways, then there is a potential for stimulating this process. One attempt to do this is presented by van Bilsen and van Emst (in Chapter 3) in their development of 'motivational interviewing' techniques, for use in working with heroin users who are considering the possibility of change. This is concerned with the skills required to engage clients, and to encourage them to return again, because services which don't see clients cannot influence them. Most chapters address this issue of engaging potential customers, and the implications of this for the organisation of services. Hamlin and Hammersley (in Chapter 7) describe the importance of first contacts with benzodiazepine users, and ways of handling these so as to maximise the possibility of engaging them in treatment. The chapter on family therapy describes ways of drawing partners and parents into this demanding treatment approach. Understanding the varying and fluctuating nature of motivation has implications for engaging and working with a wider group of drug users.

The roles of medication

Only one chapter focuses exclusively on medical treatments, but every other contribution discusses them. Pharmacological treatments fulfil a variety of functions and most treatment approaches require an integration of medical and non-medical components. Prescribing drugs can attract opiate users into contact with services so as to facilitate many of the treatments described in this book. It can help drug takers move away from injection. Users dependent on opiates can often be helped to withdraw humanely through the detoxification procedures described in detail by Choudry (in Chapter 6), just as those dependent on benzodiazepines can be helped by the prescribing strategies recommended by Hamlin and Hammersley. Helping opiate users gain access to these treatments can be a frustrating task for non-prescribing services; in Chapter 10 there is a clear description of the frustrations felt by Community Drug Teams (CDTs) working with GPs whose guidelines of practice with this group is to 'just say no'. Another area of frustration for non-prescribers lies in the primacy accorded to 'the script' by drug users, elevating it in importance to a much higher status than the personal changes that psychological procedures attempt to bring about. Ways of avoiding these conflicts include the combination of family therapy with a non-negotiable methadone regime, and low threshold prescribing programmes which facilitate constructive contact (van Bilsen and van Emst's 'motivational milieu therapy'). Some non-prescribing Community Drug Teams described by Schneider, *et al.* (in Chapter 10) have found it necessary to integrate their work with that of prescribers. The argument for integrated medical and non-medical help also comes from findings that the intensity of the opiate withdrawal syndrome is strongly affected by such psychological factors as emotionality and anxiety levels, and can be alleviated by presenting accurate information about the time course of the syndrome (Phillips, Gossop, and Bradley 1986; Green and Gossop 1988).

The potential for drug services to learn from elsewhere

Many of the current discussions about drug services are being conducted as if they were completely unique. During 1987 controversies about prescribing practice became widespread (as evidenced by a series of articles in *Druglink*), debating the value of maintenance prescribing. As Wilks argues in her discussion of these issues (in Chapter 9), these arguments have generally not been informed by a critical appreciation of evidence from the past. Arguments for and against, for example, the prescription of injectable heroin, have made little reference to this country's experience of carrying out such a policy in the past. Strong arguments for maintenance prescribing in Britain today have been proposed using historical evidence from other countries. For example, Marks (1987) cites Vaillant's (1973) work to argue for a ten-year natural span for heroin addiction – making the questionable assumption that this work is directly relevant to drug use in Britain today, based as it is on the experience of New York addicts detoxified in hospital in Kentucky in 1953. Services can learn from a critical reading of the past, and also from the experiences of other services. Clement argues in her review of issues arising in other community teams, particularly Community Alcohol Teams (CATs), that few of the dilemmas faced by CDTs are entirely new (Chapter 11). In many districts CDTs are the very first service for drug takers and have responded to novel problems in creative ways (see Chapter 10). Yet many of their management and policy issues have been already faced by CATs and Community Mental Handicap Teams, and ignoring the lessons learned there may prove foolhardy.

These four issues reflect changes and developments in attempts to respond to the problems of drug users, when, in the era of AIDS, the philosophy and practice of services need to be reconsidered in order to reach and serve a wider population.

References

Green, L. and Gossop, M. (1988) 'Effects of information on the opiate withdrawal syndrome', *British Journal of Addiction* 83: 305–9.

Marks, J. (1987) 'State rationed drugs', *Druglink* 2 (4): 14.

Phillips, G.T., Gossop, M., and Bradley, B. (1986) 'The influence of psychological factors on the opiate withdrawal syndrome', *British Journal of Psychiatry* 149: 235–8.

Prochaska, J.O. and DiClemente, C.C. (1984) *The Transtheoretical Approach: Crossing Traditional Boundaries of Therapy*, Homewood, Ill.: Dow-Jones-Irwin.

Vaillant, G.E. (1973) 'A twenty year follow-up of New York narcotic addicts', *Archives of General Psychiatry* 29: 237–41.

Part One

Developments in Views of Drug Abuse

Chapter Two

Changing conceptions of the nature of drug abuse

Gillian Tober

The drug-taker's tale

PJ is 21. She has just finished making a television documentary on 'heroin addiction'. Her mother, who organises a support group for the parents of drug addicts, persuaded her to do it. All it involved was telling her story – her past, her present, and how she saw the future. She remembered her childhood quite well; her mother was often away from home or intoxicated at home when she was quite small; she had a slightly older sister whom she seemed to follow through life. PJ remembers first going to school, a year after her sister had started, remembers feeling so shy and frightened of the other children she would hide under the coats in the cloakroom. She remembers her sister always being good at things – school, music, sports – she remembers wanting to be special or clever at something. Most of her school years were uncomfortable – she never seemed to know how to make friends or be friends with other people.

At the age of 13 she began listening to rock'n'roll music and then going to concerts. One day some older children from school recognised her at a concert and invited her to join them. They were smoking cannabis and offered her some. She accepted, mainly because it was what they were doing and she was flattered to be asked to join them. She enjoyed the effect of the cannabis – because it made the music sound better and made her feel more relaxed about being younger than the others. It made her feel grown-up.

From then on PJ looked out for the same group of youngsters at concerts and regularly joined them, smoked cannabis with them and had a good time. After a few months she was at a concert where her friends knew the boys in the band; they all went off to a party afterwards and PJ was invited along. At the party there were drugs other than cannabis – some white powder people were snorting off mirrors through twenty pound notes. PJ was intrigued; when offered some she immediately agreed and liked the effect. Again it made her feel confident and she chatted easily with the boys in the band. They invited her to come with them to see their concert.

Meanwhile at home and at school all was not well. PJ had started to buy her own supplies of cannabis because she reckoned she could do with feeling good – feeling warm and confident on more occasions than just at concerts. Also she did not want to be reliant on other people for supplies of cannabis but wanted to make a contribution herself. She had started to smoke cannabis at home in her room and her mother had 'caught' her at it. Feeling very guilty about an alcohol problem she once had, her mother tried to talk to PJ about the possible dangers of drug taking – rather than telling her off about it. But for PJ – if this was dangerous then she would put up with the risks. She was having a great time, she had friends, she was accepted. At school, rather than just being shy and isolated, she now had a secret world she could dream about. When they told her not to come to school with purple make-up and a ring in her nostril she felt secretly proud. Before she had only felt embarrassed when she was told off for the way she looked – her uncombed hair or dirty fingernails. She was embarrassed because it drew attention to her elf-like figure.

The more PJ took drugs at parties and concerts, the more the days in between seemed bleak and empty, and the more she wanted to improve them by having her own supplies. She would rush home from school to smoke some cannabis and thereafter have a pleasant evening. PJ's mother was getting increasingly worried about PJ's drug taking and confided in the family doctor, who subsequently had a talk with PJ. He told her she would have to become a 'common whore' to support her drug taking – and she may well become one anyway if she hung around with rock'n'roll bands. This was not how PJ saw herself.

Becoming increasingly alienated from family, school and other people in positions of authority, PJ sought out her drug-taking friends more and more for comfort, affirmation and affection. When she was eventually introduced to heroin she reckoned she had discovered the drug that satisfied her need for all those things – all she had to do was get hold of it.

PJ was 17 when first she was offered heroin. She had tried most other drugs, amphetamine, cocaine, cannabis, LSD and barbiturates. The only drug she had felt inclined to take regularly was cannabis. It had a reliably comforting effect even if it did occasionally seem to cause some anxiety and morbid fantasies. But heroin was different from anything else. She just felt good, without the anxiety and paranoia. She preferred it to the other drugs. Moreover, if she injected it (and injecting drugs was not new to her as she had done this with amphetamine and barbiturates) she would get a sensation to begin with that made her feel completely wonderful. The others told her that sex was like this. With heroin she would never have to let anyone look at her body, or so she thought then.

'For there is nothing good or bad but thinking makes it so'

PJ has learned to take drugs. Her early drug taking was a response to *internal triggers* (the desire to be accepted by a particular group of people), and *external triggers* (the drug-taking habits of that particular group of people). The consequences of her drug taking were, as she perceived them, that she came to be accepted by that group of people, and additionally, that she enjoyed the effects of the drugs. She felt more relaxed, less self-conscious, and subsequently warm and loved, these *positive consequences* encouraged her to continue to take drugs. The expectation of relaxation and acceptance came to operate as triggers or *cues* for drug taking at particular times of the day and week, in other words – the consequences of the drug taking became cues for drug taking – when PJ felt to be in need of relaxation and/or social contact. Certainly there were some negative consequences like trouble with the family and family doctor and difficulties at school, but these negative consequences were *less important* to her and they were also *less immediate*.

This process of learning a behaviour by the consequences of that behaviour is called operant conditioning or instrumental learning. It is described fully in relation to problem drinking by Heather and Robertson (1985), and it is quite easy to see the parallels with drug taking.

The important feature about the consequences of PJ's drug taking is that the desired, or positive, consequences came *first*, the negative consequences were less immediate, often quite delayed. They were also of less importance to PJ than acceptance by the desired peer group and the feeling of well-being most usually experienced with her drug taking. This behaviour was therefore reinforced by its positive consequences. It is a common psychological principle that the consequences following *most immediately* after the behaviour have the more potent effect on that behaviour than consequences that are delayed. This principle accounts for people doing all sorts of things which, at first glance, seem to be doing them a great deal of harm.

Positive reinforcement, as described above, occurs when the behaviour brings about immediate positive consequences and is likely to be repeated because of these. Two other sorts of reinforcement are important in the understanding of drug-taking behaviour, namely *intermittent reinforcement*, and *negative reinforcement*.

PJ's experiences with drugs were not always good; sometimes she had a 'bad trip', sometimes she did not get stoned at all if the drugs were contaminated with too many adulterants. The expected consequence does not need to occur every time in order for the behaviour to be strengthened. Gambling is the obvious example. Reinforcement that occurs only *intermittently* may be even more powerful than that which occurs every time.

Second, PJ's drug-taking behaviour is not only strengthened because of the pleasure it brings, but also because of the avoidance of pain and discomfort. It takes away the discomfort of feeling lonely or self-conscious – and as her drug taking becomes more habitual it takes away the discomfort she experiences when she has had no drugs recently. This is called negative reinforcement – the behaviour is strengthened because it *prevents* or *avoids* negative events.

This sort of reinforcement is very familiar with regular heroin users and may be the major factor in continuing the behaviour. 'I do it to feel normal', 'I feel terrible if I don't have any'. Similarly with problem drinkers. *Relief drinking* refers to drinking that is designed to alleviate or avoid withdrawal symptoms; similarly, heroin users may seek regular doses of heroin in order to avoid experiencing unpleasant withdrawal symptoms. It is not the fact of experiencing withdrawal symptoms itself which encourages the behaviour; rather it is the individual's belief and experience that more of the drug will take away the symptoms or prevent them occurring, which results in a regular or dependent pattern of drug taking.

This understanding of the behaviour is essentially different from one based upon an observation of the presence or absence of the physical events (the withdrawal symptoms). What is critical is the way the individual *responds* to the presence or the anticipation of those physical events. In other words, the actual experience of withdrawal symptoms (which are, after all, the consequences of regular excessive use of a drug to which the body has become tolerant) is not as important, for the purpose of understanding drug-taking behaviour, as what the person does about the withdrawal symptoms. How does the person construe them? Are they something that will go away after a while, or is it the case that 'I can't bear this feeling and must do something to prevent it'?

In summary PJ learned to take drugs in the following way. Heroin (or any other drug) is available in particular circumstances where there is a desire for relaxation, escape or conformity with a drug-taking group. Taking the drug fulfils those desires. There are a number of undesired consequences but these are eliminated by further drug taking. PJ has learned this cause-and-effect relationship, though she may only think about it when for some reason she is prevented from taking the drug, and has a strong desire to do so.

It is useful to describe this state as one of dependence in the sense that Russell (1979) has used the term. PJ would experience difficulty in refraining from drug use – mainly because of the anticipated discomfort – physical, psychological, and social. She would lose the sense of physical well-being, lose the feeling of comfort, security, and affection, and lose access to the desired peer group. She would also lose the escape route from friction with family and school. It is true that this friction may well dissipate in the future but this would take time. The immediate consequences of stopping would be unpleasant; the positive consequences, if any, would be delayed. This makes it difficult for PJ to give up – there are no immediate positive consequences for doing so.

As PJ came toward the end of her story she noticed she was being more selective about what she told the television crew. Up to the point about taking heroin regularly it all seemed fairly reasonable; but there was more to it than how captivating the drug was. There was the need to raise money or do straight sex-for-drugs business. It was true that as long as she had an adequate supply she could remain stoned while she raised money for the next dose. But sometimes she had to do it in the cold light of day, sober or withdrawing, and experience all the humiliation not only of having sex with a stranger, but also the comments on her 'elf-like' figure. She did not tell them any of that. She did tell them that she would get drugs 'on tick' and then they'd come round and threaten her for the money; when she had money they would press her to buy drugs she didn't want. She told them about other things she minded – her father throwing her out, having to live alone in a bedsitter, not having money for the electricity bill, being cold when the supply was cut off. She minded that her mother thought it was all her fault. When she began to cry the producer asked: 'Why don't you see someone about it?' 'There's no point,' she said, 'they'll only tell me to stop and I can't at the moment.'

To continue to understand how PJ's behaviour is affected not only by its consequences, but by PJ's perception of those consequences – what has happened eventually is that the balance, described earlier, between negative and positive consequences, is changing.

Sometimes this changing balance occurs abruptly, for example, with an arrest, or a particularly bad drug experience. Sometimes it will be a gradually occurring process – the experience of negative

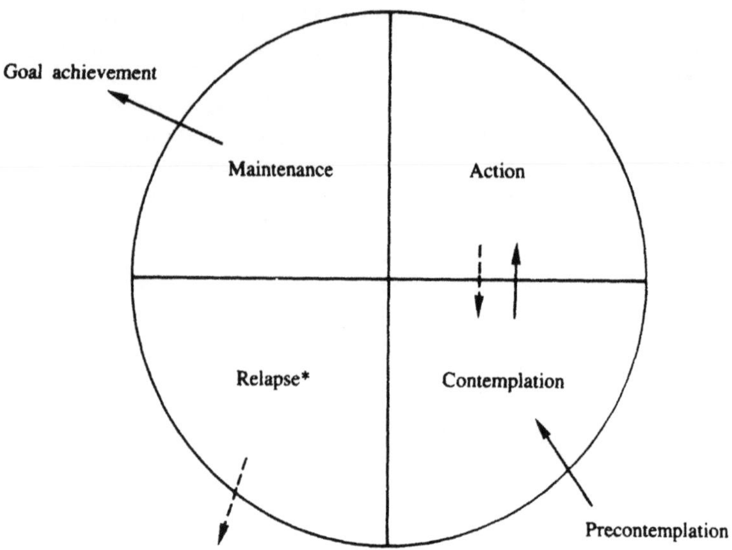

* Drug-taking episodes may occur at any stage and are not to be confused with relapse

Figure 2.1 The model of change

Source: Adapted from Prochaska and DiClemente 1984

consequences increases while the experience of positive consequences diminishes. For PJ, having to trade her body for drugs detracts from her 'craving' for warmth and human affection; the warmth and affection of her family is becoming more and more distant and inaccessible – she is beginning to think that perhaps she could have the latter at a much lower price than the warmth afforded her by the heroin.

This shift in the balance of consequences – the negative consequences come to outweigh the positive consequences – they become more immediate and more important – creates conflict about the behaviour. Sometimes the conflict will endure – on the one hand some of the consequences are unacceptable, but on the other hand, 'I can't live without it', or, 'I don't believe I can give it up'. Alternatively the individual may resolve the conflict very quickly. This may be done either by giving up the problem behaviour itself, or by changing the thoughts that create the conflict. Thus PJ may stop taking heroin, return to the bosom of her family and try to live happily ever after. But she may resolve the conflict by saying, 'Oh well, plenty of girls work for a living, it's not so bad, it's what you have to do when you're a junkie'.

Prochaska and DiClemente (1984) have described this state of conflict as being characteristic of the first stage in the cycle of change. Their model (see Figure 2.1) is useful in distinguishing the stages of change an individual goes through in his or her attempts to give up/gain control over a problem behaviour.

Before the making of the television programme, PJ could be described as a *precontemplator*. A precontemplator's thoughts characteristically rationalise the problem behaviour (if the individual thinks about it at all), for example, 'It's not a problem for me', or, 'There's nothing I can do about it'. The precontemplator selectively attends to the positive consequences of the behaviour and plays down the negative consequences, or finds ways of resolving these. In substance misuse a repetition of the behaviour itself will often alleviate its negative consequences. PJ, for example, would use drugs in order to feel better, and her drug-taking activities would take her out of the house and away from the friction with her parents (as well as being at the root of this friction).

At the time of making the television programme PJ is beginning to move into the *contemplation* stage; this stage is characterised by feelings of conflict about her drug-taking behaviour. On the one hand PJ is 'hooked' on the good things she gets out of taking heroin, but on the other hand she is getting frightened. What she has to do to get the heroin is becoming increasingly abhorrent to her. Increasingly she experiences a mixture of good and bad results; a couple of times she has become quite ill from injecting contaminated materials, or has immediately regretted using a needle and syringe that has been used by other people. She knows about AIDS. One of the parents in her mother's support group had a son who died of it.

So when the producer rings her up two weeks later to say he has found someone who will see her and discuss some options with her, she decides to go along.

A lot of the people we see in our agencies are 'precontemplators'; they are there because someone has 'made' them come. This may be a magistrate or judge, a spouse or parent, an employer. Coming to the agency may assist in eliminating any potential conflict – it enables people to say 'it can't be *that* bad now because I'm doing something about it'. Equally they may come because they want to resolve a different problem: the threat of imprisonment, homelessness, marital breakdown, job loss. These factors are described by Prochaska and DiClemente (1984) as being different *levels* of potential change, and they have an important role to play in the resolution of the substance misuse problem.

Some people recognise their substance misuse as a problem: 'I'm drinking too much', 'My drug taking is out of control'. This is referred to as a problem at the substance misuse level. Others recognise problems in their relationships with others – 'My wife has threatened to leave me'. This is an example of problems at the interpersonal level. Another level is described as the intrapersonal level – 'I feel depressed/anxious all the time'. Problems with the law, housing problems, employment difficulties, are described as problems at the social systems level. It is often the case that individuals approach agencies for help with problems at these other levels and are motivated to change behaviour in order to resolve these problems. It will be the task of the helping agent to harness this motivation to change by developing a recognition of the connection between the presenting problem and the substance misuse problem.

'There is no one for whom we cannot do something'

The advantage of having a theoretical framework for understanding drug taking and related behaviours is that it can be applied equally to an understanding of how the individual changes or gives up these behaviours, and as such must provide the basis for planning intervention strategies. The rest of the chapter is devoted to illustrating the application of this understanding of drug-taking behaviour and change.

The ultimate goal in seeing PJ may be to get her to stop using drugs. But at this stage of her drug-taking career it is important just to see her, and there is plenty to be done before she is ready to give up. She can reduce the amount of harm she is doing and reduce the number of risks she takes; she needs to experience greater conflict about her drug taking before she reaches a decision to stop. This greater conflict has traditionally been seen as resulting from the maximum amount of drug-related suffering – the 'rock bottom' effect. But equally she can experience greater conflict through accumulating rewards for a behaviour which conflicts with the drug-taking behaviour: coming to the clinic regularly and enjoying a warm and caring attitude from medical staff and others in positions of authority, having people take a concerned (rather than dismissive) interest in her drug taking, the possibility of taking drugs in a controlled and sterile manner – drugs which will reduce the effect of heroin if she continues to take it. In other words she might begin to see the benefit of changing her behaviour.

When the conflict becomes intolerable and there is no escape route through rationalising away the negative consequences, PJ is likely to reach a decision to change her drug-taking behaviour. This decision will indicate a move into the next stage of change, the *action* stage. It is in this stage that a behavioural change occurs – either giving up the drug-taking behaviour or imposing controls upon it. This behavioural change consists of unlearning previous responses (taking heroin in response to triggers in given situations) and learning new responses to those triggers. It is accompanied by a belief in one's ability to make these changes. PJ will have to learn new responses to the invitations of friends to parties and concerts where drugs will be offered to her. Furthermore she will have to discover new sources of acceptance, warmth and human affection. These tasks are accomplished in the *maintenance stage* of change, the stage during which the behaviour change is consolidated and maintained. If she fails to find new sources of reward she may relapse into the old behaviour. If on the other hand she does find new sources of reward for her needs she will gain confidence in remaining drug free, and the riskiness of feeling the need for acceptance, warmth, and so on will diminish.

Identifying the stage of change an individual is at is essential for deciding upon appropriate goals and the means of attaining these goals. Ignoring the different stages of change often results in the offer of identical and usually inappropriate interventions to individuals with very different needs.

How then can this model of change be used to inform our decisions about the appropriate interventions?

Precontemplation

Precontemplators are traditionally described as people who are 'not motivated'. This statement is a moral judgement not an objective one. It means 'not motivated to do what I want them to do which is to stop taking drugs'. In fact, precontemplators are highly motivated, but they are motivated to continue in their behaviour, not to change it.

Two broad categories of interventions are appropriate with precontemplators – damage limitation strategies, and motivational change strategies. Nor are they mutually exclusive. Marks (1987) has argued that a great deal of damage will be prevented by prescribing clean drugs and, furthermore, by developing a positive relationship between user and therapeutic agent in the process. Parry (1987) has shown how this positive relationship, created by a needle and syringe exchange scheme, can result in a motivational change. The opportunity to experience the benefits of less hazardous drug use, a less chaotic life-style, and a positive relationship with a therapeutic agent, have resulted in a positive perception of the possibility of behaviour change and precipitated a move into the contemplation stage.

The list of possible damage limitation strategies is as long as the list of harms resulting from problem drug use. In addition to the above examples, it could include periods of hospitalisation or equivalent asylum to facilitate a temporary drug-free state and eliminate some of the fear of withdrawal, vitamin supplements to individuals suffering the consequences of nutritional deficiencies, or food and shelter for the homeless. Berger (1987) has described a project that aims to provide housing for excessive drinkers who are precontemplators, that is, continuing to drink, and initiatives of this kind may well be applied in the field of drug abuse.

Interventions aimed at limiting the damage to families and offspring of problem drinkers may have got out of hand in the United States where spouses and offspring are deemed to have the disease 'co-dependence' or 'co-alcoholism' themselves (Miller 1987), for which hospitalisation is often recommended, but the catalogue of harms accruing to family members is suggestive of a far greater variety of remedial interventions than simply removing the children or otherwise isolating the family member with the drug-taking problem.

The reason for suggesting that damage limitation and motivational change strategies are not mutually exclusive is as follows: where people experience improvement in one area of their lives they are likely to seek further improvement in other areas. From a behavioural perspective, where behaviour change is rewarded, the expectation of reward is likely to generalise to other behaviour changes. This is the 'success breeds success' principle. The converse of this principle is that failure tends to produce the expectation of further failure.

Motivational change is often brought about by naturally occurring events which may be beyond our power to affect. The death of a close friend or relative from lung cancer will often cause an individual to reconsider his own smoking. Some life events will not precipitate change because they are not construed as being related to the drug-taking behaviour. For example, when M died of AIDS PJ could have said to herself, 'He got it while he was in the Merchant Navy – all those ports in Africa'. Or she could have said, 'Well, that means never share needles. If I have a clean set of works I'll be OK'. But instead she said, 'No matter how many clean works I have, there could always be a time when I'd use someone else's'. Miller (1983) has shown how counsellors can assist clients to come to these conclusions themselves in relation to problem drinking. His principles of motivational interviewing are applicable to change in all sorts of problem behaviours. They are described more fully by Henck van Bilsen and Andree van Emst in Chapter 3.

Sovereign and Miller (1987) have also shown the importance of *optimism* as a therapist characteristic that is associated with good outcome. It is helpful in promoting optimism to remember that maturing out of drug use is a naturally occurring process. Winick (1962) has described this process with opiate drug users in the United States, and his findings are borne out by the consistently low numbers of opiate drug users, aged forty years or more, identified in prevalence studies in the UK.

The fact that change will occur naturally, and indeed can be precipitated, is a strong argument in favour of limiting the damage while misuse continues.

Contemplation

In the contemplation stage further motivational work needs to be done; as PJ said, she is not ready to give up her drug taking. She is in conflict about it, but she is not convinced that the negative consequences of taking heroin outweigh the positive ones. She is not convinced that she will be able to do without it, that she will not suffer a lot without it.

One of the critical points in Miller's (1983) motivational techniques is that the client has to arrive at his or her own definition of the problem. It is the individual's *own* experience of a problem, not someone *else* saying it's a problem, which motivates towards behaviour change. His techniques may not be new but they provide a refreshing restatement of good (that is, useful, effective) counselling techniques. An accusing attitude will only provoke defence (commonly called 'denial' or 'lying' in the addictions field) and will be counterproductive. Miller (1983) argues for the efficacy of eliciting information and thoughts about the behaviour from the client, and he has shown the effect of giving objective (as opposed to subjective) feedback on factual information produced by the client in the Drinker's Check-Up (Miller *et al.* 1988). Again, these principles are readily adaptable to the problem of drug abuse.

There is an abundance of questionnaires, monitoring forms, diaries, and decision matrices available for use with people in the contemplation stage of change. These instruments assist the client in recording as factually and extensively as possible the nature of the behaviour and all of its consequences. For example, the client is asked to record in exactly what circumstances does the behaviour occur: when, where, with whom, what thoughts, feelings, moods are present. The client is then asked to record the whole range of consequences, the positive, negative, short term and long term.

The objective at this stage is to bring about a motivational change by *increasing* the conflict the individual experiences about the behaviour. The worse PJ feels about her drug taking and the more *possible* the idea of giving it up, the more likely she is to want to change it. Interventions in the contemplation stage will therefore be designed to bring the individual to a *decision* to change the behaviour.

Action

Once the decision to change the behaviour has been made – then it is appropriate to embark upon behavioural and environmental change interventions.

In order to change a behaviour that has been very well learned – or 'overlearned' as is the case in dependent behaviour (where the response to triggers is virtually 'automatic', that is, the individual thinks more about *how* to do it than *whether* to do it) – it may be necessary to monitor carefully the circumstances in which the behaviour occurs first. Where the major circumstances are the experience or anticipation of withdrawal symptoms, for example, it is possible to eliminate the trigger for drug taking by detoxification, prescribing the drug or a preferable alternative in sufficient quantities to prevent withdrawal symptoms occurring. It is important to recognise that withdrawal symptoms are rarely the sole trigger; the need for relaxation, oblivion, excitement, acceptance by a peer group, will not be removed by detoxification. Other strategies must be used to deal with these triggers. The need for relaxation may be met with alternative relaxation techniques, or by removal of the need, for example, removal of the source of anxiety, stress, etc. Hodgson and Miller (1982) describe the variety of self-management strategies designed to bring a problem behaviour under control by identifying the circumstances in which the behaviour occurs (self-monitoring), and either changing or eliminating the circumstances (cue avoidance) or learning different responses to them (cue exposure). These principles have been utilised in the development of self-help manuals (Blenheim Project 1982; Robertson and Heather 1986), which are particularly useful where individuals do not wish to attend an agency or are unable to do so.

Colin Brewer *et al.* (1988) have described the efficacy of using a pharmacological agent which renders heroin ineffective. If used at the action stage, administration of this preparation will change the user's expectation of what will happen if he or she takes heroin. This may be a particularly useful intervention for those individuals who described an experience of 'craving', a very strong desire for the drug in circumstances where the drug was previously taken. It helps the individual to maintain the resolve to abstain in the face of strong temptations to use, by substituting the expectation that the heroin would have no effect anyway.

Maintenance

This is the stage in which change in the behaviour is consolidated, and from which the individual may exit the cycle of change to a drug-free life, or one where control over the behaviour has become the norm.

It is neither possible nor desirable to remove some triggers such as the need for excitement or acceptance by a peer group. Interventions aimed at these needs may take a substantial amount of time. They will usually involve major changes in life-style, and there is some controversy about whether they 'should' pre-date or post-date changes in the drug-taking behaviour. A very sound principle in addictions interventions is to look at what naturally occurs and to enhance and encourage the process of natural change. In this vein, Griffith Edwards (1982) likened the task of the therapist to that of the carpenter, working with the grain of the wood. In a study of heroin addicts who had become abstinent from heroin use, Wille (1983) showed that equal numbers of people made life-style changes *before* becoming drug free as did *after* becoming drug free. This finding lends support to the preference for a flexible approach which offers the possibility of both routes to recovery.

Life-style changes will decrease the likelihood that drug-taking triggers will occur in the future, and will establish new sources of reward for persisting needs. When PJ gets to this stage she will need to find comfort and affirmation from a group of non-drug-taking friends, and she will need to find different but *equally rewarding* sources of excitement and entertainment to those which revolve around drug taking.

Marlatt and Gordon (1985) have described the role of alternative positive addictions in preventing relapse during the maintenance stage. They describe alternative positive addictions as having short-term negative but long-term positive effects. The benefit of positive addictions is (1) that they usually are incompatible with the problem behaviour, for example, running and smoking; (2) they create new sources of reward, raise self-esteem and self-efficacy, and by doing this they (3) reduce the likelihood that triggers for the problem behaviour will occur. They do not teach people what to do when these triggers do occur.

Relapse

Prochaska and DiClemente (1984) have described this as the stage following on from maintenance. It is the stage people enter where they fail to maintain the changed behaviour. From it they may exit the cycle of change back to precontemplation with such thoughts as 'I knew I couldn't do it', 'I knew I was addicted', or they may re-enter the contemplation stage and proceed through the cycle once more.

It is perhaps the fact that usually more time is spent in avoiding drug-taking triggers than in learning alternative responses to them that accounts for the frequency of relapse in addictive behaviour.

Putting relapse on the map was an important move forward at a time when little attention was paid to the problems of maintaining changed behaviours, when a dose of detoxification treatment followed by more or less intensive, but still loosely defined, counselling or group therapy was deemed to be the 'treatment' for addiction problems.

Most importantly it made those post-change drug-taking episodes a legitimate focus of further or continuing intervention rather than an indication of 'failure' or 'non-compliance'. Relapse prevention programmes proliferated; more recently questions about the nature of relapse have emerged. Saunders and Allsop (1987) have reviewed definitions of relapse, and Rankin (1988) has questioned the validity of using the term at all. Until the individual has learned new responses to drug-taking triggers rather than merely having learned to avoid them, it cannot legitimately be said that he or she has unlearned the problem behaviour. In Chapter 5, relapse prevention training is described by Mike Scott.

Take PJ: 12 months later she is attending an Addiction Unit regularly. She receives 40 milligrams of methadone a day. She has moved into a little council flat, which she likes, in a different town. She has injected heroin on four occasions during the past year and each occasion has been a single dose. She has stopped going to concerts and cut off contact with her former drug-taking associates. She is quite lonely, but her relationship with her family is much improved and she spends a lot of time with parents, grandmother, and sister. She frequents the public library and has become interested in witchcraft.

Do her four drug-taking episodes constitute relapses? Clearly not. It is easy to see how much she has changed her life-style but how far she still has to go. To treat those episodes as relapses – perhaps to stop her methadone, or to suggest that she has failed in some way, would obviously be detrimental to her making further progress.

At this point the model of change loses its simplicity. How do we define the stage PJ is at? As far as her substance misuse goes she has made dramatic changes: she has stopped using barbiturates and 'street' heroin, stopped injecting, and prostitution. She feels much more in control of her life. She is far from abstinent from opioid drugs and continues to believe that she cannot live without them. PJ with her previous chaotic life-style was in the highest risk category of 'drug addicts'; she is now in the lowest risk category. She is a 'stable addict' (Stimson and Oppenheimer 1984). Her health and social circumstances are much improved. She will continue to explore alternative activities, alternative sources of interest and satisfaction, and these will reduce the likelihood of high-risk situations occurring. But the problem that continues to thwart her, and us, is – Saturday evening, alone in her flat, a knock on the door, and Fred and Sheila come in: 'We've got some really ace gear – want to try some?'

Strategies for dealing with these situations – when the triggers for drug taking threaten to overwhelm the individual – have been described and shown to be effective by Allsop *et al.* (1987) in relation to problem drinking. These strategies encompass individually tailored, highly detailed, cognitive and behavioural control measures. Similar strategies are described by Rankin (1982) and the Sobells (1978), and by Robertson and Heather (1986), all in relation to problem drinking. They are readily adaptable to the problem drug taker. They are essentially different from teaching former addicts to live in therapeutic communities, or in the drug-free environment of the hospital ward.

These interventions are designed to help the individual to un-learn the problem behaviour and replace it with new, less harmful, more appropriate behaviours. It has been argued (Rankin 1988), that this is the central and essential business of treating addictive behaviours.

Whether or not these are relapse prevention strategies or are more generally the business of un-learning dependent behaviour is possibly not a debate we have to settle here; it is, however, important to ensure that appropriate interventions are offered, and that decisions about these are based upon an accurate assessment of whether the individual has reached a decision to change or is yet to do so. Before offering interventions designed to help change behaviour and maintain the change, it will often be necessary to offer interventions designed to reduce damage and bring about a motivational change.

Summary

Although social learning theory is not as new or controversial in the drugs field as it is in the alcohol field, it has too frequently been abandoned in the design of service delivery. Often at the point where interventions are offered to people with problems of drug misuse, theory is replaced by morally motivated statements about what the individual 'should' do. This switch results in the offer of a very limited range of interventions to a very small number of people for whom they may be of use.

Adopting a social learning approach in the context of the 'transtheoretical' model of change not only provides an understanding of addiction behaviour which accounts for the observed phenomena, it also informs and directs responses to produce a wide variety of interventions which are able to meet the demands of the whole spectrum of drug problems rather than the very select few currently catered for.

References

Allsop, S., Saunders, W., and McNamee, B. (1987) *Relapse Prevention Management with Problem Drinkers: The Results of a Controlled Trial*, Paper presented at the 7th International Conference on Alcohol Problems, Liverpool.

Berger, S. (1987) 'A humane approach to housing', *Alcohol Concern*, 3: 17–18 (May/June).

Blenheim Project (1982) *How to Stop (A Do-It-Yourself Guide to Opiate Withdrawal)*, London: Blenheim Project.

Brewer, C., Rezae, H., and Bailey, C. (1988) 'Opioid Withdrawal and naltrexone induction in 48–72 hours with minimal drop-out, using a modification of the Naltrexone-clonidine technique', *British Journal of Psychiatry*, 153: 340–3.

Edwards, G. (1982) *The Treatment of Drinking Problems: A Guide to Helping Professions*, London: Grant McIntyre.

Heather, N. (1986) 'Minimal treatment interventions for problem drinkers', in G. Edwards (ed.) *Current Issues in Clinical Psychology*, London: Plenum.

Heather, N. and Robertson, I. (1985) *Problem Drinking: The New Approach*, Harmondsworth: Penguin Books.

Hodgson, R. and Miller, P. (1982) *Self-watching: Addictions, Habits, Compulsions: What to do about them*, New York: Century Publishing Co.

Marks, J. (1987) 'State rationed drugs', *Druglink*, 2 (4): 14.

Marlatt, G.A. and Gordon, J.R. (1985) *Relapse Prevention*, New York: Guilford Press, pp. 299–300.

Miller, W.R. (1983) 'Motivational interviewing with problem drinkers', *Behavioural Psychotherapy*, 11: 147–72.

Miller, W.R. (1987) 'Cousins of Alcoholics', *Psychology of Addictive Behaviours* I: 74–6.

Miller, W.R., Sovereign, R.G., and Krege, B. (1988) 'Motivational Interviewing with problem drinkers: II The Drinker's Check-up as a preventive intervention', *Behavioural Psychotherapy*, 16: 251–68.

Parry, A. (1987) 'Needle swop in Mersey', *Druglink*, 2 (1): 7.

Prochaska, J.O. and DiClemente, C.C. (1984) *The Transtheoretical Approach: Crossing Traditional Boundaries of Therapy*, Homewood, Ill.: Dow-Jones-Irwin.

Rankin, H. (1982) 'Cue exposure in South London', in N. Hay and P. Nathan (eds) *Clinical Cases in the Behaviour Treatment of Alcoholism*, New York: Plenum Press.

Rankin, H. (1988) 'Relapse and eating disorders: the recurring illusion', in M. Gossop (ed.) *Relapse and Addictive Behaviour*, London: Croom Helm.

Robertson, I. and Heather, N. (1986) *Let's drink to your health*, Leicester: British Psychological Society.

Russell, M.A.H. (1979) 'What is dependence?', in G. Edwards, M.A. Hawks, and M.D. MacCafferty (eds) *Drugs and Drug Dependence*, London: Saxon House, Lexington Books.

Saunders, B. and Allsop, S. (1987) 'Relapse: A psychological perspective', *British Journal of Addiction*, 82: 417–429.

Sobell, M.B. and Sobell, L.C. (1978) *Behavioural Treatment of Alcohol Problems*, New York: Plenum Press.

Sovereign, R.G. and Miller, W.R. (1987) *Effects of therapist style on resistance and outcome among problem drinkers*. Paper presented at the International Conference on the Treatment of Addictive Behaviours (ICTAB), Bergen, Norway.

Stimson, G.V. and Oppenheimer, E. (1984) *Heroin Addiction*, London: Tavistock.

Wille, R. (1983) 'Processes of recovery from heroin dependence: relationship to treatment, social changes and drug use', *Journal of Drug Issues*, 13: 333–42.

Winick, C. (1962) 'Maturing out of narcotic addiction', *Bulletin on Narcotics*, 14: 1–7.

Part Two

Developments in Treatment

Chapter Three

Motivating heroin users for change

Henck van Bilsen and Andree van Emst

Why do we need motivational interviewing techniques?

Heroin addicts, heroin users, and other people suffering from addictions are often in the stages of precontemplation or contemplation (see Chapter 2 in this book). Before it is worthwhile starting a treatment programme, the clients have to reach the stage of active change, and once they have reached this stage (Prochaska and DiClemente 1984) a fair number of change-directed therapeutic procedures are available (Miller 1980). In other words, in order to benefit from treatment the client has to be motivated. It is possible to support the transition from the stage of contemplation to the stage of active change, if appropriate therapeutic interventions are applied.

A goal of the motivational interviewing approach should therefore be to stimulate and to supervise the contemplation and decision-making of the client concerning his 'problem' behaviour so that he takes into consideration all the relevant pros and cons of change and non-change. Such a task has consequences for the attitudes of the therapist and for the nature of the therapeutic interventions. In this approach the client himself is seen to be responsible for his behaviour and the problems. The therapist has to accept this and should not have inflexible ideas abut the decisions a client should make. A moralising attitude cannot pass muster. Contact between client and therapist should be directed towards raising the self-efficacy and self-esteem of the client. It is helpful for the therapist to view himself as someone who guides clients through the dangerous land of decision-making. It is his task to stimulate the client into starting an internal re-evaluation of his situation in such a way, that it leads to a 'wise' (all pros and cons considered) decision. The therapist tries to create an atmosphere in which the client motivates himself. The client can only motivate himself if he becomes more aware of his behaviour and the nature and seriousness of the consequences of that behaviour. He also has to become more clearly aware of the motives for his behaviour, potential contradictions within it, and the possibilities for change.

Motivational interviewing techniques

Motivation interventions

The most important motivational interventions are (van Bilsen 1986a, 1986b, 1987; Miller, 1983, 1985; van Bilsen, van Emst, and Schippers 1986):

1. Creating an empathic atmosphere of unconditional positive regard for the client.
2. Giving the client clear and concrete feedback about his behaviour, motives and personal situation.
3. Structuring and providing choice alternatives concerning the addictive behaviour and the problems.
4. Staying in contact with the client.
5. Actively listening to the client.

To carry out motivational interviewing, therapists require a wide repertoire of therapeutic skills. They must be able to use reflective, provocative, and directive interventions, to empathise with the client, but also utilise restructuring when required. Clinical success comes from using these skills in a flexible, integrated, manner.

Motivational techniques

During motivational interviewing the therapist makes use of the above mentioned interventions. Putting these interventions to practical use means employing several techniques:

Reflecting what the client says

Utterances of the client signifying motivation are reinforced. This can be done by empathic repetition of what the client has said. The therapist tries to select and emphasise these statements in which the client expresses motivation in the direction of change. By doing this the therapist stimulates the client to express more of these 'self-motivational' statements. The therapist can reflect what the client says at different 'levels', ranging from a mere literal repetition of the words spoken by the client to a reflection of the client's feelings (underneath the spoken words). The former are mostly used in the beginning of a motivational process (see 'eliciting phase'), and the latter are used when the therapist feels that he has begun forming a therapeutic relationship with the client.

Examples of reflections:

Client: Sometimes I feel anxious, thinking of all my wasted years. Will I ever be able to lead a normal life?
Therapist: You are really worried about your future, aren't you?
Client: I don't know. Sometimes I really want to stop leading this life, but what's in store for me if I stop using heroin?
Therapist: You have many doubts whether it is worthwhile for you to stop using heroin.

Structuring

It is very important that the therapist brings structure to the information the client is giving. It is helpful to reorganise all the information the client provides in such a manner that it gives the client a deeper understanding of his own (psychological, social, emotional, and medical) circumstances. The therapist can structure the things the client says by making lists on a black-board or flip chart. For instance, a week's drug use can be written down 'just to get the picture, so you can decide for yourself whether your boyfriend is justly worried about your drug use'. A similar approach can be used in giving the client feedback on his medical situation after a medical check-up. This structuring is done in an empathic non-moralising manner. The facts are not presented in a confrontative way ('Your health is already bad, if you go on using that stuff you'll surely die'), but in a low key fashion ('As you can see on the medical chart, your liver has been damaged, some of this damage is irreversible, most of it could recover').

Restructuring

Restructuring, or positive labelling of experiences and utterances of the client, is used to provide a different, more positive, meaning for the client's experiences, behaviour or feelings. If clients have predominantly negative views of their experiences, behaviours or feelings, then the use of restructuring by the therapist creates a more positive interpretation for them. The therapist helps the client to construe events more positively – an important process in the development of self-esteem and self-efficacy expectations.

Examples of restructuring:

Client: I have been using heroin almost all my life, I have rows with my family, I have debts everywhere. I have a jail sentence hanging over me, so I woke up this morning and said to myself: 'let's get some therapy', and here I am. What do you want me to do?

Therapist: You seem to be a vigorous person. You have already made a list of all your problems and you are willing to do something about them!

Or

Client: I know what this so called therapy is all about, it is a kind of brainwashing; you won't trick me into this kind of junk.

Therapist: You seem to be a very critical person, you have definite ideas about the way you don't want to change your life; could you tell me a bit more about these ideas?

Summarising

When the client is talking to the therapist, one type of structuring is so important that it requires special attention. During sessions a therapist can give brief summaries of what the client has said. Sometimes it is necessary to summarise very often, after each utterance of the client. It is always good to give a few summaries during the session, just to sum up everything the client has said, in order to check whether the therapist has understood correctly, and also to provide the client with feedback on the things he has said.

Asking questions

Questioning can be a valuable technique. By asking the right questions at the correct moments the therapist can help the client to be much more concrete and specific in the things that he says. The therapist can phrase questions in certain ways in order to help the client provide information which is as concrete as possible. This is most important when the therapist is making an inventory of client's drug use.

Example of asking questions:

Client: O.K., let's try and make an inventory of my drug use, but mind you, I have a very bad memory.

DO NOT ASK:

Therapist: Let's start last Monday. Did you use drugs on Monday morning?

BUT ASK INSTEAD:

Therapist: Let's start on last Monday. Could you tell me how much heroin you used on Monday morning, say between 8 a.m. and 1 p.m.?

Provoking

Provoking, or the use of paradox, is a special way of eliciting statements from the client. The therapist takes the role of the devil's advocate. He plays the part of denial to elicit from the client statements signifying the opposite. With this method the therapist 'seduces' a client into the role of proving to the therapist that there are problems, and that change is necessary.

Example of provoking:

Client: I don't have that many problems because of my drug use!

Therapist: Yes, that's my idea exactly, you don't use that much, you almost have no problems at all. Why should you want to change something?

Client: But sometimes I really get fed up with all the drug hassle.

Phases of motivational interviewing

In the process of motivational interviewing three phases can be distinguished (van Emst, van Bilsen, and Schippers 1984):

The eliciting phase

The task of the therapist in this first phase of motivational interviewing is to elicit self-motivational statements. This is based on the principle of attribution: you believe what you hear yourself say. Self-motivational statements are utterances of the client indicating awareness of drug-related problems (cognition) and/or concern about these problems (emotional) and/or acknowledgement of the necessity to change the addicted life-style (behaviour). During the eliciting phase the therapist tries to motivate the client at least to come back for another session and to establish a kind of minimal contact with the client. As it is, the therapist must receive permission from the client to be allowed to 'meddle' with the client's life. The eliciting phase can be short (one session) or very long. The more the contact between therapist and client is perceived by the client as mandatory, the longer the eliciting phase will last.

The information phase

During this phase, the client has become a bit curious about his personal situation ('Perhaps it is worthwhile to chat with this bloke, at least he doesn't preach to me!'). The therapist has seduced the client into giving permission to the therapist to ask questions in order to give the client an overview of his life and possible problems. Client and therapist start an active quest for information. It is very important that client as well as therapist find it useful and necessary to gather all this information. The therapist often has to achieve an agreement with the client on this through negotiation. With the assistance of the information that is gathered the client can decide whether there are enough reasons to be concerned about his situation. The therapist makes an inventory of the information in all possible problem areas (social, medical, and psychological). This information is fed back to the client in a neutral, low key fashion so that he gets a better understanding of his situation. It is of the utmost importance that all the information is provided in a neutral way so that the client himself draws conclusions from it. The task of the therapist remains that of coaching the client in his decision-making process. The therapist does not accept that he should be the one to prove that this client has problems or that change is necessary for this client. On the contrary, the therapist will again play the devil's advocate (provoking): 'Is it really that bad, that change is the only alternative?', or, 'You enjoy being with your friends in the drug scene, why should you give up their fine companionship for the hard clean world?' The therapist collects information and feeds this back in a neutral manner to the client. This could include, among other aspects: the amount of drug use (presented in terms of amount of money during the year/month/length of addiction), facts about his health, social, and psychological situation. The therapist always leaves the client with the responsibility of drawing conclusions from the facts.

The negotiation phase

A third phase consists of the negotiation between therapist and client. By the end of the information phase a client should have made a decision: 'Do I want to continue or do I want change?' (note: the therapist has to value both decisions equally: it may be a wise decision of the client not to want change!). It is equally important that the therapist does not have strong and outspoken opinions on how the client should change. The client has to decide whether change should be achieved, also what kind of change, and by which change strategy is he going to change. These are all the client's decisions. If a client has decided to change (for instance to decrease his heroin use from seven times a week to once a week) then in this phase the therapist's task is to give the client information on the possible treatment goals (pros and cons of abstinence and controlled use) and the treatment methods available. In doing this, the therapist takes care that the client gets good information. On the basis of this information the client is in a position to make an informed choice about the treatment goal and methods.

Practical application of motivational interviewing techniques with drug abusers

Introduction

Motivational interviewing techniques can only be applied when the therapist is in contact with drug abusers: without contact there can be no influence. It is valuable for those professionals who regularly come into contact with drug abusers to be able to utilise these techniques. Doctors, nurses, social workers, and probation officers, who come into contact with, and need to engage, drug takers, would benefit from training in this approach. It is also important for treatment agencies to create an optimum number of interactions between staff and clients. If you never see a client you can hardly motivate them. Depending on facilities and resources, a drug treatment agency can set up a 'motivational structure'. This requires a means of bringing clients and staff into frequent constructive contact: two ways of doing this are needle-exchange schemes and the prescription of methadone.

The Motivational Milieu Therapy (MMT)

The MMT is an example of motivational structure connected with the prescription of methadone that has been created by several treatment agencies in the Netherlands.

Precontemplation and contemplation

Giving methadone to heroin addicts is a common practice in the Netherlands. A traditional outpatient methadone clinic is based on the traditional treatment philosophy described in Table 3.1. The client receives methadone on a daily schedule, often together with mandatory counselling. Until the end of 1982 our clinic worked in this way, but several experiences led us to reconsider our programme:

(a) The staff spent a lot of time arguing and disputing with the clients rather than building up therapeutic relationships with them.

Table 3.1 The traditional treatment philosophy versus motivational interviewing

Motivational interviewing	*Traditional approach*
Denial/telling lies	
• Denial and telling lies are seen as an interpersonal behaviour pattern (communication) influenced by the interviewer's behaviour.	• Denial and telling lies are seen as a personal trait of the heroin addict/junky, requiring heavy confrontation by the interviewer
• Lies and denial are met with reflections.	• Lies and denial are met with argument/correction.
Labelling	
• There is a general de-emphasis on labels. Confessions of being a junky or being an irresponsible heroin addict are seen as irrelevant.	• There is a heavy emphasis on acceptance of the person as a junky or an addict.
• Objective data of impairment are presented in a low-key fashion, not imposing any conclusion on the client.	• Objective data of impairment are presented in confrontive fashion; as proof of a progressive disease and the necessity of complete abstinence.
Individual responsibility	
• Emphasis on personal choice regarding future use of heroin.	• Emphasis on the disease of addiction which reduces personal choice.
• Goal of treatment is negotiated, based on data and preferences.	• The treatment goal is always total and lifelong abstinence.
• Controlled heroin use is a possible goal though not optimal for all.	• Controlled heroin use is dismissed as impossible.
Internal attribution	
• The individual is not seen as able to control and choose.	• The individual is seen as helpless towards heroin and unable to control his/her own heroin use.
• The interviewer focuses on eliciting the client's own statement of concern regarding the heroin use.	• The interviewer presents perceived evidence to convince the client of his or her problem.

(b) The clients were not half as eager to change their addicted life-style as the therapists.
(c) There were a large number of burn-out casualties among the staff, and a large number of drop-outs from the clients.
(d) The clients were very dissatisfied with our treatment programme.

While we were contemplating our treatment philosophy, we also realised that we had a very peculiar way of thinking about addictive behaviour problems, compared with other psychological problems. Perhaps an example might clarify this. Suppose, for instance, we have treated a client with severe agoraphobia who had not dared to leave her own home. Six months after the end of treatment this client tells us, in a follow-up session, that she does not need further treatment though she still suffers occasionally from anxiety attacks and does not leave her house on dark nights. What would we conclude? This is a relatively successful case, the client is satisfied and so are we! Let's take another example. We have treated a heroin addict. Six months after the end of treatment he comes to us in a follow-up session; he tells us that he is very content with the treatment he has received. He feels he has solved his addiction problems, although he still uses heroin once or twice a week and sometimes a bit of cocaine. What would we conclude? This client has been cheating us, why didn't he come back for additional treatment when he relapsed? The client disagrees with us, he does not feel he has relapsed, he feels he controls his drug use. We feel disappointed: 'You can't trust these junkies!'

Heroin addiction seems to elicit from the therapist a huge amount of concern, so much concern, that there is nothing left for the client!

Two facts were very clear to us whilst we were contemplating change in our clinic:

(e) The clients had to come to the clinic five days a week; this could offer an excellent opportunity to influence clients.
(f) Participating in a methadone programme does not mean that this person is also motivated to change his addicted life-style.

Decision

After some time spent in the contemplation stage we arrived at two worthwhile options for change:

1. Developing selection methods, in order to treat only clients who are motivated for our treatment.
2. Developing a technique to motivate clients for change.

We decided to choose the second option.

During that period we had discovered William Miller's ideas on motivation in relation to alcohol problems (Miller 1983). We decided to try to develop these ideas, in such a way that they would also be applicable for heroin addicts.

Active change

We developed our present MMT ideas during that period. Heroin addiction and heroin use were no longer looked upon as signs of an underlying disease. Consequently, heroin addicts are not seen as suffering from a disease that must be cured. Heroin use and heroin addiction are now seen as learned behaviours, that have a high risk of creating problems for those who engage in them. Heroin addicts and heroin users in our present society run a high risk of damaging their own lives and the lives of others. We see the prevention of damage as the primary goal of the treatment for heroin addiction.

Consequently, the MMT tries to give heroin users and heroin addicts a chance to learn survival skills that enable them to live the life they want to lead with the least possible damage, to themselves and other people:

The basic attitudes of MMT

The basic attitude of MMT is humanistic. The key principles of the MMT are:

(a) Accepting the client as he is in a complete and unconditional way.
(b) Leaving all responsibility with the client for drug use and the problems connected with it.
(c) Treating the client as a grown-up responsible person, capable of making his own decisions.
(d) Waiting until the client has committed himself to the goal of change and the change strategy before starting therapy aiming at change.
(e) Negotiating the goal and strategy of treatment with the client.

The major differences between the MMT and the traditional/moralising/confrontational method are summarised in Table 3.1.

The MMT programme

All the clients in the MMT apply originally for the prescription of methadone. Most clients have to come to the clinic every day to collect their methadone. Clients are allowed to come to the clinic during a specified hour, every day, and about fifteen clients come during that time. We try to provide a motivational milieu in which these visits to the clinic can take place. In order to receive their methadone, clients have to pass through a space furnished like a living room and they can sit, talk, drink coffee/tea for an hour here every day. Two staff members are always present; one, a nurse, in the separate methadone delivery room, and the other, a social worker, in the MMT room. These try to create the motivational milieu atmosphere. Their most important task is to use motivational interviewing skills (van Bilsen 1986a) in order to create a friendly empathic atmosphere. Staff encourage, elicit, and introduce discussions on topics of importance to the group (for example, troubles with the rising price of heroin, worries about AIDS, and so on). The staff also ensure that the general rules are followed by all the participants so that a steady, stable, and safe atmosphere is created. In this relaxed, open, and permissive climate, the staff always treat the clients as adults who are responsible for themselves. The staff 'diagnose' which stage of change each client is in and develop motivation plans accordingly. The goal of the interventions of the therapists is to motivate the clients to move from precontemplation to decision. The staff pinpoint certain desired behaviours for each client and, whenever possible, they try to put these behaviours into a contingency reinforcement schedule.

An example might clarify the need for creativity in the process of pinpointing desired behaviours. It concerns a very shy, small heroin addict whose only interaction with other people was complaining. Some days he went on complaining to another client or a staff member for the whole MMT hour. His complaints were about his health, his heroin use, and so on. We wanted him to look upon himself in a more positive way. We started by analysing exactly what he did during the MMT hours and discovered that he sometimes (once a week) tried to tease staff members. He seemed to enjoy this, although he did not receive any credit for it. We started reinforcing this action of his by giving him attention whenever he did it, praised him for his teasing qualities in front of other clients, and so on. In doing this we used pinpointing of behaviour to raise the self-esteem and self-efficacy of the client.

During the daily contact between staff and clients, the staff use motivational interviewing techniques to reinforce desired behaviours, to encourage clients to speak and to keep to the rules of the MMT. Depending on the stage of change the client is in, there can be different goals: raising self-esteem (during precontemplation); eliciting self-motivational statements and developing self-efficacy (during contemplation); changing attitudes and behaviour (during action). The notion of individual responsibility is very important in dealing with the person's heroin use and methadone dose. Negotiation is a key process in these matters. The methadone dose the client receives each day is not imposed by the physician: it is arrived at by discussing the possibilities in an open atmosphere, so that, within broad limits, clients are allowed to choose their methadone dose. No direct pressure is put on the client to change his use of heroin. The client has to decide how to handle his opiate use in the future. Clients are allowed to stop their methadone intake for a few days (when they have used heroin) (van Bilsen and van Emst 1986).

There is evidence that opinions which are forced on people do not hold, while opinions reached by their own reasoning or experience do hold (Janis and Mann 1977; Prochaska and DiClemente 1984). Thus the staff do not initiate discussions about changing the addicted life-style, but, rather, reinforce clients when they start talking about it by themselves.

Some examples of motivational interventions in MMT

The three months' evaluation system

Every three months a client participating in MMT is evaluated by the staff. They collect all the material available on the client, discuss it and then decide on a strategic manner of feeding this material back to the client, often through an interview or a letter.

Writing letters to the clients

This is an important motivational tool that might be used by the staff to present the client with their observations in a low key fashion, often using a story-telling technique.

Clients are given responsibility to determine their own dose of methadone

If they have used heroin on a particular day, and then come to collect their methadone, they are given the choice as to whether to take their complete dose of methadone, or less, or none at all.

Some practical issues

What is necessary to develop motivational interviewing techniques and interventions? First of all there are tutoring, practice, and supervision. It may look easy at first sight to practise motivational interviewing, but our experience from numerous workshops and training courses in the Netherlands as well as the UK has shown us that only a small minority of therapists have these motivational skills available for systematic, unprejudiced use with their clients. Excellent training materials are available for instruction in motivational interviewing (van Bilsen, van Emst, and Schippers 1986; van Bilsen and Bennett 1987). Practising motivational interviewing techniques and interventions requires a corresponding philosophy on the part of the agency. One of the key principles is that the addict has to decide for himself what should be done (if something should be done). The policy of the agency should allow the option of the client choosing not to change, and controlled use as a negotiable treatment goal.

Possible pitfalls

Even therapists who have studied all that there is to study on motivational interviewing, have made several video tapes on the subject, and are invited to do workshops on the topic, are by no means infallible. For our own benefit, and we hope for the benefit of other therapists, we have studied our own shortcomings. The following pitfalls are the most dangerous ravines to stumble into as a therapist working with the motivational problem of addicts.

The therapist imposes the treatment goal on the client

When a client enters a treatment unit for addiction problems, there seems to be only one option for a treatment goal; complete and lifelong abstinence of the substance that was abused. This is the treatment goal we are brought up with. Often society as a whole, the spouse of the client, or the therapist who referred the client, have very clear opinions about the future use of drugs by the client: he or she should abstain completely. Often confronting the client with this therapy goal leads to disputes about its necessity. If a client starts arguing with a therapist about the treatment goal of complete and lifelong abstinence, he is likely to be labelled by the therapist as unmotivated or as a typical denying drug taker. When we work as therapists in other areas of psychological problems (for example, phobias, marital problems, social skills problems), we do accept the ideas of the client concerning the treatment goals. Why do we act differently in the field of addictions? Stating the treatment goal as a non-negotiable fact often traps the client and therapist in a maze of non-productive arguments which prevents the development of the necessary working alliance between them.

It is also a very demotivating option for therapists. As a therapist you will never see a treatment success if your definition of this is the client who remains completely abstinent, no longer commits any criminal activities, and has a legal job for the rest of his life. Clients as well as therapists profit from stating realistic, workable, attainable, and, above all, negotiable, treatment goals.

Starting with change-directed interventions without having reached an explicit agreement with the client

The basis for every behaviour therapy is a functional analysis. This should be a theory about the problem behaviour of the client, which should be shared with the client and with which the client has to agree. How often have you as a therapist started treatment without doing this? And how often were you then disappointed in the motivation of your client to bring about changes?

It looks as if therapists in the field of addictions (and also behaviour therapists) are afraid to discuss the theories and ideas that they develop on the problems of the clients with the clients themselves. The client who intends entering treatment, in order to keep his job by cutting down his drinking habit, may not be at all motivated to stop drinking, nor to discuss with the therapist his marital problems that cause his drinking (according to the therapist). Our therapist, however, is again strengthened in his belief, that all alcoholics are denying their real problems and are unmotivated to stop drinking.

Not being able as a therapist to do without reinforcements from the progress of the clients

Psychotherapy with addicts rarely provides us with the rapid successes of which we, as therapists, have been dreaming. Heroin addicts tend not to be very grateful, and a large number relapse after therapy: doing psychotherapy with them has little intrinsic reinforcement. A therapist who depends on such reinforcements will feel the need for them very soon. He might begin to lose belief in his therapeutic qualities or, equally bad, may develop a belief system in which he attributes the lack of success to the personality characteristics of the clients (for example, 'nobody can succeed with these pathological clients, these addicts have built in resistances against treatment', and so on).

Believing that addicts are unable to change

Believing that 'once an addict, always an addict' does not encourage us to believe in change. If a therapist – consciously or unconsciously – believes this, he will infect his clients with these beliefs. And if clients start believing such ideas, this will lead to the next self-fulfilling prophecy.

Accusing the clients of their problems

Treating people with addictive problems often provokes confrontations with the morals, values, and belief systems of therapists themselves. Addicts to legal and illegal drugs often do things that a therapist personally disapproves of.

In such a way therapists often are seduced into letting the client know their disapproval of her prostitution or of his driving while intoxicated. In our opinion it is not the task of the therapist to make moral judgements about the client. On the contrary, it is the task of the therapist to raise the client's self-esteem, to give him the feeling that he is accepted as a person by the therapist despite his or her human weaknesses. The basic attitude of a therapist should be one of accepting what is, rather than of demanding what should be.

Too quick, too radical, therapeutic interventions

People with addictive problems are often able, in many ways, to influence themselves and their therapists into feeling that right now there is an urgent need for somebody (i.e. the therapist) to do something. Action is needed in order to rescue the client. The client hands the responsibility of the problems over to the therapist. Therapists are seduced into asking their clients to change something. This can vary widely: asking a client to stop drinking in the evenings, or getting the client into in-patient treatment. Often therapists defend their radical interventions with a statement such as: 'I could not let this . . . [terrible thing] happen to my client'. These therapists are over involved with the pain their patients feel; this therapist is not a therapist any more, but a worried parent.

Results

The value of motivational interviewing as an effective tool in motivating problem drug users for behaviour change remains to be established. Elements of motivational interviewing (for example, empathic listening, providing choices, and so on) have a positive effect on the therapy success rate, but the approach has not yet been thoroughly researched (Miller 1983; Miller and Schippers 1983; Miller 1985). Our own experience is limited to the Motivational Milieu Therapy in our own clinical practice and is, of course, biased. In our MMT a small research project was carried out from 1985 to 1987. Twenty-five clients of the MMT programme were interviewed with the Addiction Severity Index (ASI) (McLellan *et al.* 1985). We were able to interview the clients three times, at the start of the research period, three months afterwards, and again after twelve months. There was no control no-treatment group or any group receiving 'traditional' treatment. The results can only indicate change and cannot provide scientific proof that the MMT caused the change.

The Addiction Severity Index

It was difficult to find a research instrument that matched our ideas of motivation and change. The design of the ASI is based upon the premise that addiction must be considered in the context of the problems that contribute to and result from the drug abuse. The objective of the ASI is to produce a problem severity profile for each patient through an analysis of six general areas which commonly result in treatment problems (McLellan *et al.* 1985; van Bilsen 1987). These are: drug abuse, medical, psychological, legal, family/social, and employment/support. Within the ASI much attention is given to the 'need for additional treatment', as perceived by interviewer and client. For example, a client who has very poor uncorrected vision, but has been fitted with glasses which allow him to see adequately, would still be considered to have a severe vision problem if severity were defined as 'deviation from optimal function'. However, the ASI estimate would be quite low, since no additional treatment would be required. This is the major reason for our choice of the ASI as the evaluation instrument: the client's opinion of whether treatment is needed is valued highly. A severity profile is built from the client's severity rating, the severity rating of the therapist and some objective facts.

Some results

The clients

Their average age was 28.3 years, their length of drug use was 12.4 years. The average client is a male caucasian, in his late twenties, unemployed, living on his own, who got into drugs during his adolescence and who has lived most of his life in the area.

The severity profiles

When we look into the change of the severity profiles, from the first interview to the third interview, we see an interesting pattern, as can be seen in Table 3.2.

Table 3.2 Severity ratings of ASI in MMT

Problem severity rating	*Change of severity*	
	After 3 months	*After 12 months*
Medical	−20	−65
Employment	−25	−60
Alcohol	−60	−50
Drugs	0	−25
Legal	−20	−90
Family	−50	−50
Psychological	+30	−40

Some case examples

Case 1

The client is a 22-year-old woman who had started using heroin at 14 years of age as a kind of 'self-medication' for an eating problem (*Anorexia nervosa*). She participated in the MMT for three years from the age of 18. The goals of the staff were to increase her feeling of self-esteem (by complimenting her on her clothes, and so on) and talking with her about the things she could do well), and increasing her self-efficacy. This latter involved requiring progressively more from her when she wished to receive exceptions from the MMT rules. At first she merely had to ask in order to be allowed to get methadone for a few days, but then she had to present reasons, and then good reasons, and then to discuss the soundness of her reasons with staff. The most important goal was to create a kind of attachment with the MMT. Feeling attached to the '*laissez-faire*' MMT structure gave her enough courage to start a formal psychotherapy which lasted two years. During this period she also took part in a social skills training programme. At the moment, a year after finishing with the MMT, she is doing well and leading a satisfying drug-free life.

Case 2

The client is a 26-year-old female, who had started using heroin when she was 20, influenced by her heroin-using boy friend. Despite the many interventions directed towards stimulating an alliance between her and MMT staff, we did not succeed in creating a therapeutic relationship with her. She was given a great deal of positive attention and home visits. Even when she became pregnant, she only came to the clinic three times a week. Probably her social system (her dealing, and her heroin-using boy friend) was a hindrance. She did not have enough 'room to move' to become involved in the MMT programme.

Case 3

The client is a 32-year-old male who started using heroin at the age of 18, after the death of his father, and thus escaped from the responsibilities arising within his family at that time. He participated in the MMT programme for three years. On the one hand the MMT staff thought him a very nice person, always talkative and compliant, but on the other, he was very tiring because of his complaining. The staff hypothesised that his complaints reflected essential problems and so they began to listen carefully to this complaining. This resulted in an increasing awareness in the client of his own problems (grief and depression). At the same time the client learnt that these problems could be overcome (increasing self-efficacy) so he entered therapy.

As clinicians we feel that the approaches used in these case studies and described in this chapter are promising tools to use in helping drug users develop their motivation for change. Rigorous evaluation is required to find out the extent to which these feelings are justified, and to aid the process of changing, refining, and developing our attempts to help our clients.

References

Bilsen, H.P.J.G. van (1986a) 'Motivational Milieu Therapy, motivating heroin addicts for change', Paper presented at the 15th International Institute on the Prevention and Treatment of Drug Dependence, Noordwijkerhout.

Bilsen, H.P.J.G. van (1986b) 'Moralisern of normaliseren', *Tijdschrift voor alcohol, drugs en andere psychotrope stoffen*, 12: 182–9.

Bilsen, H.P.J.G. van (1987) 'Heroin addiction; morals revisited', *Journal of substance abuse treatment*, 4: 127–34.

Bilsen, H.P.J.G. van and Bennett, G.A. (1987) *Motivational interviewing for addictive problems*, Videotape produced by East Dorset Community Drug Team.

Bilsen, H.P.J.G. van and Emst, A.J. van (1986) 'Heroin addiction and Motivational Milieu Therapy', *International Journal of the Addictions*, 21: 707–13.

Bilsen, H.P.J.G. van, Emst, A.J. van, and Schippers, G.M. (1986) *Heroine. Motivatiegesprekken met gebruikers*, K.U. Nijmegen: AV-dienst A-faculteiten.

Emst, A.J. van, Bilsen, H.P.J.G. van, and Schippers, G.M. (1984) *Ongemotiveerd. Motivatiegesprek met een probleemdrinker*, K.U. Nijmegen: AV-dienst A-faculteiten.

Janis, L. and Mann, C. (1977) *Decision making*, New York: Free Press.

McLellan, A.T., Luborsky, L., Cacciola, J., Griffith, J., Evans, F., Barr, H., and O'Brien, C.P. (1985) 'New data from the Addiction Severity Index', *Journal of Nervous and Mental Disease*, 173: 412–23.

Miller, W.R. (ed.) (1980) *The addictive behaviours: Treatment of alcoholism, drug abuse, smoking, and obesity*, Oxford: Pergamon.

Miller, W.R. (1983) 'Motivational interviewing with problem drinkers', *Behavioural Psychotherapy*, 11: 147–72.

Miller, W.R. (1985) 'Motivation for treatment: a review with special emphasis on alcoholism', *Psychological Bulletin*, 98: 84–107.

Miller, W.R. and Schippers, G.M. (1983) 'Effecten van een zelfcontroleprogramma voor probleemdrinkers', *Tijdschrift voor alcohol, drugs en andere psychotrope stoffen*, 9: 107–12.

Prochaska, J.O. and DiClemente, C.C. (1984), *The Transtheoretical Approach: Crossing Traditional Boundaries of Therapy*, Homewood, Ill.: Dow-Jones-Irwin.

Chapter Four

Family therapy and addiction

Dennis Yandoli, Geraldine Mulleady, and Claire Robbins

Introduction

Richard had been using heroin heavily for ten years. He was married and his wife did not use heroin. They had two children – three years and eight years of age. He had run into legal difficulties as a result of his heroin use and decided to refer himself to the Drug Unit. He was aware that many areas of his life had become unbearable as a result of his drug dependence. He started a methadone reduction programme, and after six months of regular counselling he had managed to successfully reduce his methadone prescription and was now drug free. He had become more confident and self reliant, starting to assert himself, and had got much more involved in the care of his children at home. Richard then decided to end his treatment.

Three months later we received a telephone call from him, distressed and confused. His wife had become seriously depressed and his eight-year-old son had become unmanageable and was refusing to go to school. Richard could no longer cope and had begun to use heroin occasionally.

Richard was yet another example of the user who was successful at coming off drugs, but whose efforts to stay drug free were undermined because we did not recognise the significance of family involvement in an individual's drug use. We began to consider the ways in which we could work with the family in order to help the user to sustain a drug-free life-style.

Why a family perspective?

Working with addicted families

During the past decade, a picture has begun to emerge which clearly points to the importance of family factors in drug addiction. This image challenges the previously held view that drug users are cut off from their families and unable to form lasting relationships. Little has been written about these families and the treatment of drug addiction. Many drug workers recognised the significance of family involvement in sustaining drug dependency without having any explicit framework for intervention. It has been firmly established that a significant proportion of drug users are not leading the chaotic, transient life-style of prolonged isolation and separation from their families, so often assumed. Vaillant (1973) looked at one hundred drug addicts in New York and found that 72 per cent of them were living with their mothers at age 22, 47 per cent by age 30. Stanton and Todd (1979) reported that of eighty-five male heroin addicts seen at the Philadelphia Veterans Drug Treatment Center, 66 per cent either resided with their parents or saw their mothers daily. Noone and Reddig (1976) found that of their 323 addicts (average age 24.4 years) 72.5 per cent either lived with their families of origin or had done so within the previous year.

These studies from the United States seemed to indicate a high percentage of drug users remaining at home, with higher percentages among younger users. In this country Fraser and Leighton (1984) showed that 38 per cent of drug users attending a Drug Dependency Unit between 26 and 30 years of age were living at home with their families. Another study by Crawley (1971) found that, of 134 opiate addicts (mean age 21) admitted to a treatment service, 52 per cent lived at home with their parents. In a five-year follow-up study, Levy (1972) found that the majority of drug addicts who responded successfully to treatment, and went on to rehabilitation, had family support. Despite possible sociocultural differences, these findings appear to cut across international boundaries.

Family relationships are more complex than the sum of the contributions of each individual, but are viewed collectively and are referred to as 'the family system'.

The purpose of family-based treatment is to focus attention on the patterns of behaviour which undermine normal efforts at leaving home and separating from the family, thus bringing about change in the client's drug use. The individual who has not separated but instead remains emotionally bound to his family can be described as 'enmeshed'.

The family functions in a way which seems to encourage or maintain the user's addiction by denying other areas of conflict within the family system (Madanes *et al.* 1980). The drug user needs to recognise their role in the family system. There is little research into this method of treatment for drug users. Stanton (1978) used a family therapy approach with adult male opiate addicts and succeeded in significantly reducing the number of days of opiate use over a period of twelve months. Haley (1980) described the function that heroin addiction can have in families – particularly where the drug use may serve to keep the family together. Del Orto (1974) found strong indications that the family system played a role in maintaining drug use. He used family participation in order to minimise the likelihood of relapse, going so far as to suggest that attempting to treat drug addicts without seeing the family was futile.

Broadly speaking, family therapists see drug addiction as having one of two consequences. The first is a distraction from other family conflicts, and the second is the avoidance of separation from the family. The most frequently cited example of this pattern of family behaviour features the addict becoming enmeshed in family life and, in the process, forgoing their own need to separate normally (Madanes *et al.* 1980).

Features of families with drug abuse

The emphasis here is on families with a member addicted to opiates. However, similar principles apply to families with other substance abuse problems.

The following features have been noted by various therapists as characteristic of the relationships and roles in families with a drug abusing member:

1. There are no clear role boundaries within the family. If one or both of the parents are drug users, then frequently the children assume a parental role. For example, an older child may take the responsibility for dressing and feeding the younger siblings, or even shopping and preparing meals for the entire family. This is often apparent, even when the children are quite young.
2. The children frequently do not experience a clear parental role from either parent. They are seen by their parents as exemplary and are often praised for their performance. Symptoms may appear in the children, frequently as difficulties in relationships with their peers.
3. Other agencies and other concerned individuals may take on the tasks of the parents. Outside agencies may assume responsibility for decision-making. Other consequences of drug use can bring unwanted inspection of the family's life-style, for example, if the drug user is arrested, a social worker may have to take action to protect the child.
4. In many families the significance of drugs is minimised by all family members, when in fact drugs may be central to the

function or dysfunction of the family.

5. Drug use has the function of maintaining the status quo or 'stuckness' of the family system; for example, in a relationship where only one partner is using drugs, drug use can serve to minimise the sexual relationship with the non-drug-using partner, and also reduce the involvement of the drug user in day-to-day living and decision-making. The drug user may potentially take on a more childlike role within the family.
6. In families where the drug user is an older adolescent or young adult, there is frequently over-involvement with the user and opposite sex parent. This is particularly true of the male user and his mother.
7. Where both partners are using drugs, often their parents disapprove of their son or daughter's chosen partner, even when the drug use predates the relationship.
8. Serious conflicts are avoided by the drug use. There is frequently a 'flatness' of emotional expression within the family. Coming off drugs involves increased conflict at all levels of family interaction. The family will often seek to prolong methadone treatment in order to avoid conflict. In cases where one member of a couple is using, the non-using spouse may feel very strongly that the therapist should prevent conflict by prescribing methadone.
9. Stanton (1979) reports that in families with a male drug user, fathers are characterised by being weak and ineffectual. Father and drug-using son frequently have a very poor relationship, and the father remains distant and withdrawn. He goes on to state that siblings of drug users often have more successful relationships with their fathers. On the other hand, fathers of female addicts are reported as inept, but indulgent and overly permissive of their daughters.
10. Death in the family often stands out as a significant feature, either as excessive grieving at the loss of a loved one, or unusual circumstances surrounding the death. There is often a shorter than usual life expectancy and a higher than normal death rate in the family. Stanton (1977) describes the unusual role addicts play in helping the family maintain stability in the face of change, including the sacrificial role of 'martyr' and 'saviour' to the family.
11. Where both partners are drug users, then the survival prospects for the relationship are better if the relationship predates the onset of drug use. If the male is providing drugs for his partner, he will be very reluctant to relinquish this role.
12. These families tend to have a rather traditional perception of

their roles as family members, for example, the drug-using father may have the role of breadwinner, even though supplying drugs may be the main source of income.

Developing a treatment model

The therapy model uses elements of both structural and strategic family therapy. Structural family therapy derives its name from the perceived importance of family composition, particularly as a hierarchy, and how this hierarchical system is organised. For example, a family with a weak and ineffectual father would be subject to an imbalance in family structure. The therapist's main objective is to identify the imbalance and to intervene by emphasising the importance of the father and his role in the family, that is, elevating his importance. Structural family therapy is widely associated with Salvador Minuchin, who used it extensively in the treatment of 'anorectic families'. Only a cursory summary is presented here. Interested readers will find these techniques covered more fully in Minuchin and Fishman (1981).

Strategic family therapy is much more concerned with how and why people change. There are many people associated with this method but Haley (1980) is the person whose work has been most widely applied to the treatment of 'addicted families'. Symptoms such as drug addiction are seen as functional in that they maintain the status quo, or 'homeostasis' of the family system. This idea is a departure from the linear view of causality and instead suggests a circular pattern where the drug user's difficulty in separating from the family is the family's way of avoiding change. The therapist attempts to intervene in a way that blocks or interrupts this cycle, and allows the family to reorganise and to adopt a more healthy response. These models are brief and intensive as well as goal oriented, and they maintain the family's involvement throughout treatment.

There is increasing evidence to support the view that drug users are dependently involved with their families, and that family factors are significant in sustaining drug use (Harbin and Maziar 1975; Klagsbrun and Davis 1977). There is also support for the view that drug users are reluctant to accept responsibility for themselves. Stanton (1979) assumes that continued drug use is rooted in the drug user's failure to disengage from the family home. For the family, having a drug-using member functions to divert attention away from their own problems. According to Haley (1980), disengagement or separation is commonly achieved when an offspring leaves home through work or school, or by establishing an intimate relationship outside the family. Some families find this period very stressful and become unstable as a result.

When the drug user is prepared to venture away from the family, he or she would start to use drugs or some other problem would develop which is synonymous with failure. This has the effect of drawing the family together in an effort to rescue the drug user. This results in stability for the family. This cycle of behaviour illustrates the family's investment in keeping the drug user dependent. Even if the drug user leaves home they have not achieved separation as long as the family is reminded of their continued drug use.

Drugs themselves seem to play a particularly effective role in facilitating this *interdependent* process where both family members and drug user remain locked or 'stuck' with one another, unable to move on to the next stage in their lives. Drugs allow the user to experience a sense of separation as well as the pleasure associated with the drugs themselves. This false separation gives the addict a sense of 'having his cake and eating it'. Drugs users also experience a false sense of separation through relationships with the drug-using subculture which supports the illusion that they have an independent life.

Family therapy in practice

Initial treatment phase

Engaging the family

Those thinking of starting a family therapy programme would be wise to question the client at referral about their willingness to include members of their family in treatment. We have found that clients are frequently more compliant at the start of treatment and therefore the earlier the question is asked, the better the chances of gaining the clients' co-operation.

Once the client has been assessed and is stable on their prescribed methadone dose, the attention should then be placed on arranging an appointment to include the rest of the family. It is sometimes necessary to hold several preliminary sessions with the client individually, in order to gain their final acceptance and co-operation when inviting the family to attend. Throughout these preliminary sessions the therapist should avoid engaging the client in discussion about treatment issues. This is necessary if the therapist is to avoid becoming alienated from the rest of the family. Our experience suggests that the therapist contact the parents directly rather than leave it to the user. It can be useful to telephone the parents at a time when the addict is with the therapist. If this is not possible, a letter should be sent to the parents, emphasising the importance of the family's involvement regardless of previous attempts to help.

Couples with one user are sometimes easier to engage in the treatment. The non-using partner can often be helpful in getting other members of the drug user's family to attend. Occasionally this causes problems, when the parents are condemning of the non-using partner.

The non-using partner is excluded from the family sessions in these cases until, with the help of therapy, the couple accept that the responsibility for drug use exists with the drug user and not with their partner. Concurrent with these sessions, the drug user and their partner will be seen together, focusing on plans for the future and relationship issues.

Couples where both partners are using drugs pose a much more difficult problem when attempting to engage one or both sets of parents. The couple frequently have a very stable relationship which maintains the false separation between themselves and their respective families. The therapist will need to focus on involving one set of parents at a time, the choice of which can be negotiated between the couple. Our experience has shown that when either partner involves their family, this poses a significant threat to the other partner, often resulting in a termination of the relationship. The drug user may then rapidly return to the family home or initiate a relationship with another drug user. If the drug-using couple initiated their relationship prior to using drugs, then the relationship stands a much better chance of survival should one or both partners become drug free.

Individuals who live with their families of origin are frequently unprepared to involve their family in sessions. The client may try to convince the therapist that no one in his family has any idea that he is using drugs. The therapist will be wise to remain incredulous at these attempts for it is very rare, in our experience, that no one in the family is aware that drug use is taking place or has been attempted at some time in the past.

Assessment

In order to assess the family structure, the following techniques may be useful:

1. The therapist can start the first session by asking the drug user, 'Who is the best person to tell us about how you have been affected by your drug use?' The response can indicate an important relationship between the drug user and the identified spokesperson.
2. It is useful to spend some time discussing the details and

procedures which make up their treatment. The drug user should be encouraged to describe to the family the details of the treatment programme. Some of the issues to raise are discussion of drug usage, level of prescribed methadone dosage, and the rate of reduction. This also facilitates discussion on the logical outcome of treatment, that is, being drug free. It is also helpful to make explicit the procedures that will be employed during the sessions such as the role of the co-therapist and the use of 'home-work tasks' to the family, to carry out between sessions.

3. The therapist should encourage the drug user to openly discuss the history of his/her addiction:

   (a) when he/she started;
   (b) route of administration of drugs;
   (c) how the habit is funded.

   The therapy sessions should be a safe arena to discuss these frequently emotive issues. The therapist should observe and identify alliances within the family. It is useful to note any overt behaviours which are remarkable for their repetition. An example of this might be a mother who moves her seat closer to her drug-using son during the session. One particular pattern which was common to many of our families involved the ritual of cigarette lighting during or immediately following conflict or lively discussion.

4. Another useful exercise at this stage is to draw up a genogram with the family's help. The genogram is a technique used to record both genetic and interpersonal family-household data. This frequently reveals bits of previously undisclosed history, and is remarkable for turning up drug problems in other family members such as problem drinking or tranquilliser use (see Figure 4.1, p. 60).

The therapy

Starting therapy

As the family becomes more familiar with the therapist and the clinic, they are more likely to express their genuine thoughts and feelings to the drug user. Sessions should focus on the 'degree of concern' that the family feels for the addict's behaviour, despite the fact that the statements being made about the drug user are often quite condemning and confrontative. Stanton and Todd (1982) call this 'ascribing noble intentions' in an effort to remove whatever sense of blame may cloud these sessions. It is essential to maintain a productive atmosphere in which possibility for change is explored. In doing so, it can be helpful to use statements to the drug user such as, 'It is natural for you to *protect* your family from the anxiety caused by your drug use', or to a parent, 'As a concerned parent you have made a great *sacrifice* to understand this problem'. This also serves to reduce the guilt which sustains the 'stuckness' so common with these families.

Methadone has the effect of reducing the crisis that led the drug user to seek treatment. This frequently resulted in a 'lull' in the content of the sessions after one or two appointments. During this initial phase, the family often develops a false sense of optimism regarding the drug user's ability to remain drug free, the so called 'Pink Cloud' period. The therapist should point out their familiarity with this phase of treatment and predict problems ahead, and the possible resumption of drug use as treatment progresses. The therapist may wish to preface this statement by equating these predictions with those of the character from Greek Mythology – Cassandra – a harbinger of doom and gloom who was not listened to. At this stage of treatment it is necessary to establish with the family that the treatment goal is abstinence.

Urine testing is useful in order to monitor progress, to confirm drug use; it should be made clear from the outset that there will be regular urine checks and that the results of these will be accepted as valid.

Second phase

Homework tasks

In families consisting of a drug user and both parents, it is important to get the user involved with the parent of the same sex. One way of achieving this is to negotiate specific home-work tasks which should be undertaken by both of them, for example, father and son – setting time aside to discuss the ways in which the son might cope with the problems of living a drug-free life-style. These might include coping with boredom, seeking employment, or developing wider social interests. At this stage the therapist may need to assuage the anxiety of the opposite sex parent who may feel threatened by being excluded from these tasks. Statements addressed to the opposite sex parent such as, 'They really do need to talk, don't they?' or, 'They haven't spent much time together before have they?' can be helpful in reducing this anxiety.

Conjoint and network therapy

In some cases it was impossible to engage the family in treatment.

In this situation, rather than using the co-therapist as an observer in the adjacent room, we included them in the session. They take an active role in the session and refer to the therapist as part of the system. The co-therapist takes on the role of 'live' consultant and gives direct advice to the therapist on how to run the session. This technique has been used previously by Skynner (1979).

The crisis phase

The next significant stage in the treatment is characterised by a marked change in the drug user's status, with respect to drug use. The drug user may curtail his or her illicit drug use, detoxify at home, or enter an in-patient detoxification centre. Often, this change is accompanied by a family crisis which may entail an escalation in parental/marital conflict, serious injury to a member of the family, another member revealing a drug problem, or, ironically, the family may choose this time to reject the drug user. The function of such a crisis is to undermine the drug user's efforts at separation, which the change in the drug use represents. This is an important stage in therapy, marked by the drug user achieving a degree of self support and success apart from the family. As the user's behaviour is pushing towards becoming more normal, the family may be threatened and become unstable. The crisis most commonly involves the parents' marital relationship. In one such case, after their son had entered a detoxification facility and went on to rehabilitation, the parents began to express dissatisfaction with their relationship, finding more and more fault with one another, and eventually talked of divorce. At this point the drug user learned that his parents were near to separation. This was a signal for him to relapse in order to distract the family from their disturbing marital problems by focusing once again on him instead. The crisis is the crucial point in treatment. The therapist has predicted the problem and now needs to devote considerable effort to assist the family to cope with their crisis without sabotaging the drug user's progress. The goal is to encourage the drug user to remain separate from the crisis and encourage the family to support the drug user.

Families can be quite ingenious at finding ways of manufacturing a crisis. By predicting the likelihood of the family becoming disturbed by the drug user's change in status, the therapist is attempting to defuse the destructive potential of the crisis when it occurs. Such a prediction also has the effect of enhancing the therapist's expertise. This enables him to encourage the family to use coping strategies in order to break the previous cycle of interdependency. In the example above, the therapist would encourage the family to discuss how they can prevent themselves from drawing their son back into their lives. Where appropriate, it may be useful to direct the parents to marital counselling. It is most important that the therapist help the user to continue to remain separate and persevere with his efforts to achieve independence. If the crisis fails to dislodge the user from his progress then the therapist has succeeded in breaking the recurrent pattern. Real change has occurred. It is now possible to negotiate a new set of goals in addition to maintaining abstinence, that is, the drug user's un/employment, housing, social relationships, and so on. In order to facilitate this, the therapist may choose to see the parents/drug user/partner separately. Above all, if the parents or other members of the family say that they are having serious problems and need help, the therapist must make it clear that the priority is the drug user's return to normal functioning. The same principles apply when working with couples who are both using. Should one of them begin to reduce their drug-taking behaviour, then their partner will manufacture a crisis in an effort to sabotage their progress, for example, having an overdose or getting arrested. Under these circumstances it may be appropriate to include various network personnel as members of the client's system – a probation officer, social worker, health visitor, or GP, and so on. These individuals often have an influential role in the drug user's life, and thus replicate the struggle for separation and independence that the drug user has not achieved with their parents. The drug-using couple can thus re-enact their hopelessly rebellious stance with these people of authority.

Couples – one user

An advantage of working with couples where there is a non-drug user is that the non-user can act as a role model. It has been our experience that this family configuration frequently includes children. The non-using partner often finds reduction of the methadone dosage quite threatening, and asks the therapist to increase or maintain the level of prescribed drugs. Such requests are quite common and indicate a fear that, once the user becomes drug free, underlying conflicts will rise to the surface. These conflicts will threaten the structure of the 'marital' relationship. The view most commonly held, of this marital system, is one which represents the drug user maintaining an 'extramarital affair' through illicit drug use, which his partner has tolerated in a mutual pact of denial and avoidance. The therapist, at this point, needs to cool down the emotional intensity related to the role that drugs play between the couple. The goal here is to help the couple to acknowledge the reality of drug use and to explore the prospect of change together. We recommend that the couple be encouraged to attend Families Anonymous and Narcotics Anonymous respectively as part of a 'home-work task' (Berenson 1979).

Berenson (1979) states that the purpose of this task is to establish support for themselves so that the emotional intensity is at least partially diverted from the sessions themselves. A crucial point in working with this marital system is reached when either partner begins to focus on themselves and starts to accept responsibility for perpetuating the situation.

Future treatment

It needs to be made clear time and again that responsibility for possible resumption of drug use lies solely with the recovering user. It should also be made clear that treatment can be resumed should the need arise. When the need for such sessions have arisen, it was our experience that the family was approaching a new milestone, that is, a retirement, a death, birth or marriage, and the process of generating a crisis was once again activated. Such sessions need to redefine the family boundaries, which in a crisis may appear to be crumbling.

The St. Mary's family therapy project

We decided to evaluate the efficacy of family therapy as a treatment at St. Mary's Drug Dependency Clinic. The evaluation took the form of a comparative treatment study. Clients referring themselves to the Drug Dependency Unit were asked if they were prepared to include members of their family in their treatment. If they said 'yes', then they were included in the study. A family was defined as a relative(s) from the family of origin or partner. In some cases where family participation was not possible, very close (non-drug-using) friends were included. It was evident that there were three configurations of family make-up; couples where both partners used drugs, couples with only one partner using and individual users who were residing with their family of origin or were in close contact with them.

The three configurations were labelled:

- Couples – both users.
- Couples – one user.
- Individuals – plus family of origin.

Each of the three family configurations were allocated equally to three treatment conditions:

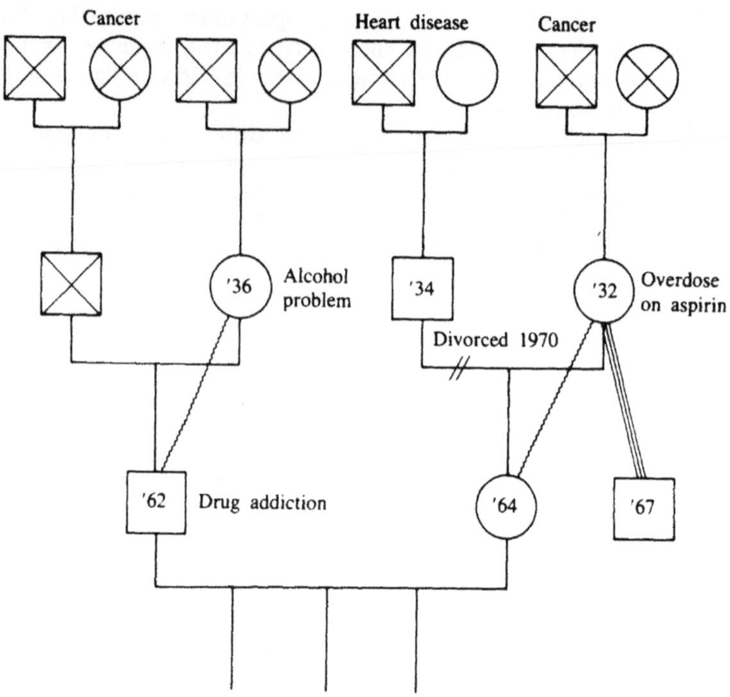

Note: The above diagram depicts several generations with sex, birth, and death rates and major interaction between several members of the household. Included are relationships which are hostile, distant, discordant and enmeshment (Jolly *et al.* 1980).

Figure 4.1 An example of a genogram

Family therapy.
Minimal contact.
Standard clinic treatment.

Family therapy (FT)

Those in this condition were prescribed methadone on a fixed reduction schedule (5 mg reduction every two weeks). Therapy consisted of brief intensive sessions with initial emphasis on engaging the family in the treatment programme. The theoretical approach of our therapy derived from both a structural and strategic model, described earlier.

Minimal contact

In this condition patients were prescribed methadone on the same fixed reduction schedule as those receiving family therapy. They also received a package of information containing relevant leaflets and various key services such as emergency housing, social security, self-help groups and legal advice. Thereafter they were seen on a monthly basis. A standard interview was then administered which reviewed their progress. The therapist would advise the client of any services which they might need or find helpful.

Standard clinic treatment

Individuals in this group were seen within the normal context of the clinic's treatment procedures and practice. The methadone programme consists of a prescribed dosage of oral methadone established following a full assessment. This includes a personal history and several urine tests. The methadone dosage (maximum 60 mg) is reduced on a flexible basis over a period of time. During the programme clients are offered regular supportive psychotherapy sessions.

Assessment battery

Prior to commencing a methadone programme, the drug user has completed an assessment battery. This used to assess changes over several areas of functioning. It included:

Research consent form

Next of kin, whether next of kin knows about drug use or not, whether we identify ourselves as DDU or not in communications with the next of kin.

Addiction Severity Index

The mainstay of our outcome measures. A relatively brief structured interview designed to provide information about aspects of the person's life which may contribute to their drug problem. This was developed in the USA (McClellan *et al.* 1980) and has been widely used there. It covers medical status, education, employment, finance and support, drug and alcohol use, legal, family, social, and psychological history. We have also added information about syringe sharing.

Tyrer anxiety scale

Brief clinical interview dealing with anxiety symptoms (Tyrer *et al.* 1984).

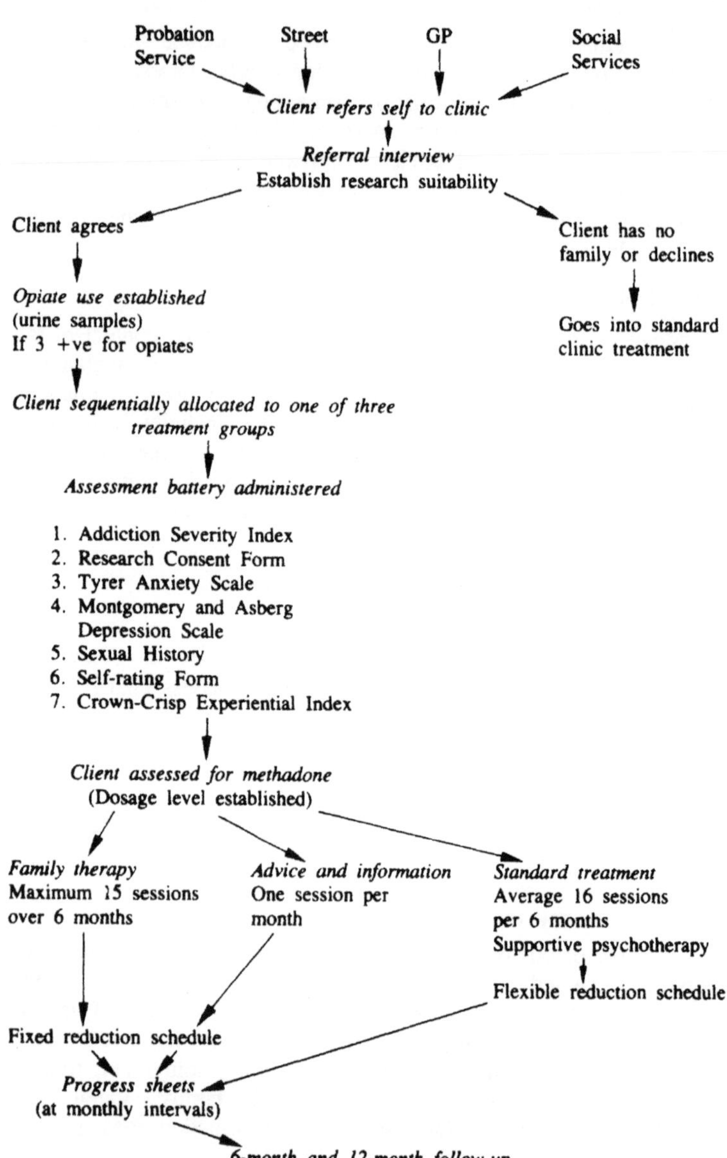

Figure 4.2 Family therapy project research design

Montgomery and Asberg depression scale

A brief clinical interview covering the symptoms of depression (Montgomery and Asberg 1979).

Sexual history

Sexual problems related to heroin abuse and how much these bother the drug user.

Self-rating form

The client rates himself on a five-point scale for anxiety, depression, dependence, coping with life, relationships with family, leisure activities, and confidence.

Crown–Crisp experiential index

A self-rating scale which gives a profile of psychological state, diagnostic information and personality (Crown and Crisp 1979).

Following completion of this assessment, clients entered the methadone programme. The average dosage of methadone was 40 mg (range 10–70 mg). The assessment battery was readministered to all three treatment groups at six- and twelve-monthly intervals from the start of treatment. One hundred and nineteen drug users took part (sixty-five men and forty-four women). In terms of family configuration there were sixty-three couples – both users, thirty-three couples – one user, and twenty-three individuals plus family of origin.

Two therapists acted as a team, one working with the family while the other viewed and taped sessions. Both therapists had prior training in family therapy. It was intended that all families should be videoed for the purpose of supervision. Out of forty-one families, only three refused to be videoed. The average number of family sessions was six per family. Supervision for the team was provided by Dr Chris Dare, a family therapist from the Maudsley Hospital. On a monthly basis supervision took place in the form of reviewing taped sessions with occasional live supervision. A significant difference between the methadone reduction schedule for this group and the standard clinic group was the rigid reduction of 5 mg every two weeks. This was considered essential in order to avoid endless and time-consuming negotiations about the reduction rate during the therapy sessions. Therapy therefore concentrated on the families' plans to assist the drug user to become drug free.

Preliminary results

The detailed analysis of the outcome is as yet incomplete. However, preliminary examination of the results does indicate a significant

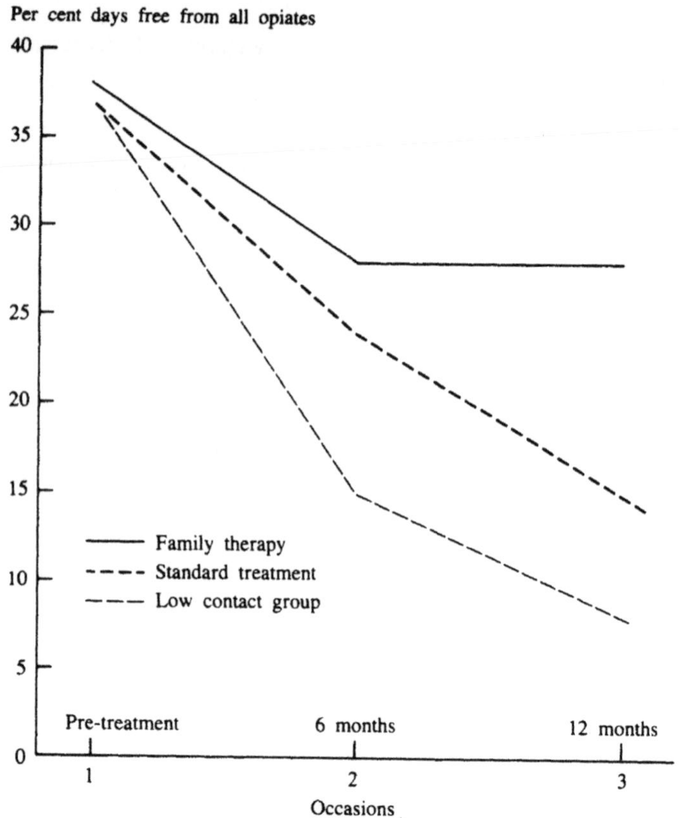

Figure 4.3 Treatment outcome: drug-free days

difference in the outcome measures between family therapy (FT), standard clinic treatment (ST), and minimal contact (MC). Significant reductions in drug use were obtained for all three treatment conditions over a twelve-month period. However, those in the family therapy treatment condition show a greater percentage of days free from heroin than the other two conditions – that is, at six months – FT 50 per cent, ST 42.5 per cent, and MC 30.5 per cent, and at twelve months – FT 28 per cent, ST 14 per cent, and MC 14 per cent. The proportions not taking any opiates (including methadone) were at six-month follow-up – FT 28 per cent, ST 24 per cent, MC

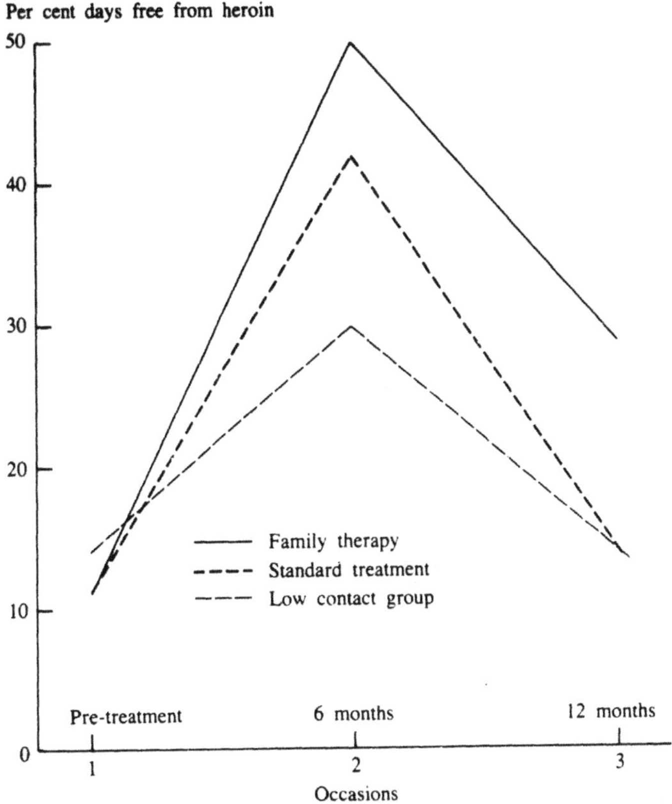

Figure 4.4 Treatment outcome: heroin-free days

15 per cent, and at twelve months – FT 28 per cent, ST 14 per cent, MC 8 per cent. The detailed further analysis will be published elsewhere but, at this point, we are able to state that family therapy is effective in reducing drug misuse.

Conclusion

The purpose of this chapter has been to offer drug workers some basic guidelines on the family treatment of drug abuse. This way of working does have implications for the therapist and for any agency that decides to use it. It requires the therapist and the agency to have a much broader perspective than usual on the nature of drug use. It can be threatening to have to face a whole family rather than an individual, and your work is more open to the scrutiny of other workers. The approach flies in the face of a traditional treatment model which identifies the drug user alone as the focus of the problem. There are therefore significant organisational changes involved if this way of working is to be adopted, for example, review of intake procedures, modification of assessment of the drug user, appropriateness of treatment, and allocation of adequate time for mutual staff supervision. Although this approach may seem daunting at first, in our experience we have found it both a worthwhile challenge and an invaluable tool in our treatment repertoire for drug users.

References

Berenson, D. (1979) 'The therapist's relationship with couples with an alcoholic member', in E. Kaufman (ed.) *Family Therapy of Drug and Alcohol Abuse*, New York: Gardner Press.

Crawley, J.A. (1971) 'A case note study of 134 outpatient drug addicts over a 17 month period', *British Journal of Addiction*, 66: 209–18.

Crown, S. and Crisp, A.H. (1979) *Manual of the Crown-Crisp Experiential Index*, London: Hodder & Stoughton.

Del Orto, A. (1974) 'The role and resources of the family during the rehabilitation process', *Journal of Psychedelic Drugs*, 6: 435–45.

Fraser, A. and Leighton, K.M. (1984) 'Characteristics of attenders at a Scottish drug dependence clinic, *British Journal of Psychiatry*, 144: 307–10.

Haley, J. (1980) *Leaving Home: Therapy with Disturbed Young People*, New York: McGraw-Hill.

Harbin, H.T. and Maziar, H.M. (1975) 'The families of drug abusers: a literature review', *Family Process*, 14: 411–31.

Jolly, W., Froom, J., and Rosen, M.G. (1980) 'The genogram', *Journal of Family Practice*, 10: 251–5.

Klagsbrun, M. and Davis, D.I. (1977) 'Substance abuse and family interaction', *Family Process*, 16: 149–73.

Levy, B. (1972) 'Five years after: a follow up of fifty narcotic addicts', *American Journal of Psychiatry*, 7: 102–6.

McLellan, A.T., Luborsky, L., Woody, G.E., and O'Brien, C.P. (1980) 'An improved diagnostic evaluation instrument for substance abuse patients: the Addiction Severity Index', *Journal of Nervous and Mental Disease*, 168: 26–33.

Madanes, C., Dukes, J., and Harbin, H. (1980), 'Family ties of heroin addicts', *Archives of General Psychiatry*, 37: 889–94.

Minuchin, S. and Fishman, C.H. (1981) *Family Therapy Techniques*, Cambridge, Mass: Harvard University Press.

Montgomery, S. and Asberg, M. (1979) 'A new depression scale designed to be sensitive to change', *British Journal of Psychiatry*, 134: 382–9.

Noone, R.J. and Reddig, R.L. (1976), 'Case studies in the family's treatment of drug abuse', *Family Process*, 15: 325–32.

Skynner, R.A.C. (1979) 'Reflections on the family therapist as family scapegoat', *Journal of Family Therapy*, 1: 7–22.

Stanton, M.D. (1972), 'Drug use in Vietnam: a survey among army personnel in two northern corps', *Archives of General Psychiatry*, 26: 270–86.

Stanton, M.D. (1977) 'The addict as Saviour: heroin, death and the family', *Family Process*, 16: 191–7.

Stanton, M.D. (1978) 'Some outcome results and aspects of structural family therapy with drug addicts', in Smith, D., Anderson, S., Buxton M., Chung, T., Gottlieb, N., and Harvey, W. (eds) *A Multicultural View of Drug Abuse: The Proceedings of the National Drug Abuse Conference – 1977*, Cambridge, Mass: Hall/Schenkman.

Stanton, M.D. (1979) 'Drugs and the family: a review of the literature', *Marriage and Family Review*, 2 (1): 1–10.

Stanton, M.D. and Todd, T.C. (1979) 'Structural family therapy with heroin addicts', in P. Kaufmann (ed.) *The Family Therapy of Drug and Alcohol Abusers*, New York: Gardner Press Inc.

Stanton, M.D. and Todd, T.C. (1982) *The Family Therapy of Drug Abuse and Addiction*, New York: The Guilford Press.

Tyrer, P., Owen, R.T., and Ciccheiti, D.V. (1984) 'The brief scale for anxiety: a subdivision of the comprehensive psychopathological rating scale', *Journal of Neurology, Neurosurgery and Psychiatry*, 47: 970–3.

Vaillant, G.E. (1973) 'A twenty year follow-up of New York narcotic addicts', *Archives of General Psychiatry*, 29: 237–41.

Chapter Five

Relapse prevention training

Mike Scott

In most areas of life mistakes are regarded as important learning experiences. Curiously this notion has been conspicuously absent from the deliberations between people with an addiction and their therapist. Yet most of those who learn to control their addiction do so by themselves after a number of unsuccessful attempts. The key feature of a Relapse Prevention Programme (RPP) is that clients are engaged in a process of actively learning from mistakes. The therapist simply facilitates the learning – nudging the client along naturally occurring pathways. An RPP can be likened to a journey in which the client as driver has decided on the ultimate destination. The therapist simply acts as accompanying navigator. A 'successful' journey involves passage through a number of overlapping phases which broadly correspond to preparing for the journey, getting started, handling slips, managing daily hassles, the pursuit of life goals and maintaining vigilance. In this chapter each of these phases is described in turn, but they should not be thought of as following in strict sequence.

Part of the art of conducting the RPP is judging when to introduce material that might 'ordinarily' be taught later in the scheme. Continuing the metaphor of a 'journey', it would be inappropriate to introduce an RP Programme if the client refuses to go to the station (that is, the client is in what Prochaska and DiClemente, 1982, term the precontemplative stage) or if the client is simply pacing up and down the station platforms (that is, is in what Prochaska and DiClemente, 1982, term the contemplative stage). Strategies for dealing with clients in these early stages are described elsewhere in this volume by van Bilsen and van Emst and also in Scott (1989). The RPP is predicated on the assumption that the client is taking active steps to modify his addictive behaviour, RPPs can encompass almost any client goal, whether it be abstinence, controlled drinking, or switching from injecting to inhaling. A client may, for example, at the beginning of therapy be on a reducing methadone script over three weeks, with a view to total abstinence from heroin, another client may have as his drinking goal, drinking seven or eight pints just two nights a week. The same principles apply whatever the goals adopted. The RP approach is applicable across the range of addictions from heroin use to cigarette smoking, and rests on considerable research evidence (Cummings, Gordon, and Marlatt 1980) suggesting that there are important commonalities amongst the addictions – even though clearly the social pharmacological aspects of the various addictions differ markedly.

The length of an RPP will vary considerably from client to client depending on the number and severity of 'roadblocks'. Some clients may, for example, need help with problems such as depression and assertion which pre-date their addictive behaviours, and are currently serving to maintain such behaviour. Other clients may need much less help. As a rough rule of thumb, seven weekly individual sessions of forty-five minutes is usually sufficient to teach the coping skills necessary to avoid full-blown relapses. (However, a considerably longer period may be needed depending on the intractability of emotional disorders and interpersonal conflicts that may act as triggers.) Sessions are then spaced at monthly intervals of six months to consolidate learning. During the follow-up phase the therapist should ideally be able to offer the client a safety net – 'if you really get stuck between the monthly sessions, give me a ring, and we can arrange to have a chat'. The aim of the sequencing of sessions from weekly to monthly is to ensure generalisation across time. Generalisation across settings typically does not happen unless it is an integral part of an intervention programme. To this end it is advised that, where possible, the therapist and client agree to engage a non-addict relative or friend to act as quasi-therapist. This person would attend the last fifteen minutes or so of each session in the period when the session content is summarised and homework assignments are set. Should difficulties arise between sessions, the quasi-therapist is on hand to provide support and advice. The non-addict relative or friend is also usually in a better position to liaise with the addict's family than the addict himself.

Preparing for the journey

Clarification of destination is a necessary first step in an RPP – the key question is what does the client wish to attain? The therapist aligns himself with whatever goal the client wishes to pursue. The goal should not be seen as insurmountable but rather as subject to change in the light of the client's ongoing experience. In order that relatively stable goals are pursued, the therapist has to carefully check out with the client the perceived 'realism' of each goal. It is important that the chosen goals of the client are not external imports but the client's own. In a period of considerable conflict with family and the police an addict can well feel 'I had better give up: it's too much hassle'. Decisions arrived at on this basis are potentially very unstable. The therapist should adopt the role of devil's advocate and probe whether the client will be left with anything meaningful should he modify his addictive behaviour. The client should be encouraged to elaborate on any expressed anticipated positive benefits of changing his addictive behaviours. In this way positive outcome expectations are nurtured. Any client successes, to date, in modifying his addictive behaviour, should be praised to reinforce his belief in his capacity to make the journey. Though this has to be done with care, the praise should not be so lavish as to effectively preclude the client from acknowledging slips for fear of rejection by the therapist.

Before embarking on any journey it is important to know what the likely terrain will be, allowing for contingency plans to be developed. Likewise it is important to know:

(a) The situations in which the client feels he is most likely to relapse. Use may be made here of Litman *et al.*'s (1983) Relapse Precipitants Inventory. This may be usefully complemented by Corney and Clare's (1985) social questionnaire, providing a more detailed specification of clients' dissatisfactions. Exploration of 'dissatisfactions' can indicate likely triggers for addictive behaviour.

(b) The attitudes which are likely to sabotage attempts to modify addictive behaviour. Use may be made here of the Scott Drug Related Attitude Questionnaire (DRAQ). The DRAQ consists of the eighteen items below, each scored on a seven-point scale from totally agree to totally disagree:

1. I cannot be happy unless most people I know admire me.
2. If a person asks for help, it is a sign of weakness.
3. If I do not do as well as other people, it means I am an inferior human being.
4. If I slip and take drugs, it is useless to try and control myself after this.
5. If you cannot do something well, there is little point in doing it at all.
6. If I fail partly, it is as bad as being a complete failure.
7. I have got to do just what I feel.
8. If I am to be a worthwhile person, I must be truly outstanding

in at least one important respect.

9. I'm too weak to control myself.
10. To be a good, moral, worthwhile person, I must help everyone who needs it.
11. I can't go without drugs when I'm down.
12. I take drugs because nobody cares about me.
13. I cannot trust other people because they might be cruel to me.
14. Difficult issues in life are best handled by being avoided as long as possible.
15. I have nothing to look forward to.
16. Being isolated from others is bound to lead to unhappiness.
17. Other people make me take drugs.
18. I have got to have what is enjoyable now.

The focus of the RP programme is on teaching clients new coping skills for situations in which they are particularly vulnerable. The learning of such skills, it is argued, is facilitated and maintained by changes in dysfunctional drug-related attitudes.

Getting started

When the client first begins to modify his addictive behaviour, withdrawal symptoms of some description are inevitable. The client's response to early symptoms exerts a major influence over the course of the addictive behaviour. Discomfort can be made bearable if the client is helped to conceptualise the withdrawal symptoms as time limited and less than catastrophic. The therapist can begin moving clients in the direction of this reconceptualisation by asking them how long they anticipate that the withdrawal will last – 'until you're an old man with a white stick, years, months, weeks, days, how long exactly?' The more the client is pressed to be specific, the more adequate the reconceptualisation. The therapist has to be cautious at taking at face value the clients' reports of the 'awfulness' of the symptoms they are experiencing. Probes such as 'are you saying the symptoms are preventing you from doing anything at all?' can help the client put the discomfort in perspective; asking the client how he thinks his symptoms compare with others, perhaps friends who have also gone through withdrawal, enables the client to locate himself on a discomfort scale. The therapist should summarise this discussion and integrate the fact that discomfort is time limited thus: 'so at the moment you're feeling better than *X* was but worse than *Y* and *Z*; maybe we can monitor how your symptoms change, perhaps by next week you will feel more like *Y*, and the week after more like *Z*'. Monitoring the discomfort in this way can create a certain distance from it. Discussions surrounding the management of withdrawal symptoms should be summarised and encapsulated in a set of self-instructions the clients practise as a homework assignment.

The set of self-instructions are essentially an antidote to the client's low tolerance of frustration. The first step involves noting an intolerance of frustration, for example, 'There I go again, saying I can't stand going without the drug, telling myself I need it'. The second step is a challenge to this idea, for example, 'Do I really need it, in the way I need food? I might want it, but do I have to have what I want?' The third step involves a change of direction: 'Maybe I'll think about it in 10 minutes; first of all I will put my favourite music on/go for a walk/ring a friend – just play it cool'. The self-instructions should be reviewed at the following session. A common problem is that clients do not apply them early enough. Clients typically go through a sequence: 'I wouldn't mind a hit; I would like a hit; I could do with a hit; I need a hit; I have got to have a hit'. The self-instructions are at their most potent the earlier in the sequence they are applied, consequently it is important for clients to become aware of the start of the sequence and utilise the coping self-statements then.

Clients entering treatment for an addiction tend to think about their behaviour in dichotomous terms, either 'I summon up all my will power and make the change', or, 'I drink/drug my life away'. Change is usually conceptualised by the client as a once and for all event. These client conceptualisations are usually mirrored in the treatment responses, which often approximate to 'you've got to abstain, you're wrecking your life, look what it's doing to . . .' The combination of interaction with other treatment agencies and the client's standard self-talk means that they are often taken by surprise in the presentation of the rationale of Relapse Prevention. In many cases the client struggles to put the rationale in one of his two standard boxes, usually 'you're really telling me that I can go out of here and use'. The therapist response to this should be of the form 'today is Tuesday, if one of your goals is to use on Tuesdays that's fine I'll help you achieve it'. It's not uncommon for clients to report feeling 'scary' at this point, often for the first time responsibility is being placed squarely on the client for his addictive behaviour. The client may resist this by replying 'if you tell me not to use this week I won't because you've asked me'. An appropriate therapist response would be of the form 'Why should I give you the same advice as other people? Their advice didn't work for you or you would not be sitting here now'.

The therapist should not be unduly alarmed if between presentation of the RP rationale and the next session the client has a slip.

This is often an important learning point, that along with the apparent increased freedom of the RP Programme goes responsibility. Client *A* illustrates this. He was pursuing a goal of controlled drinking, his target was seven or eight pints on a Friday and Saturday night. The session after presenting RP rationale he arrived crestfallen. He reported that he had messed up the week. Closer examination revealed that he had got very drunk on the Tuesday. The therapist asked him: 'Do you think it would be a more realistic goal to drink on Tuesday as well as on Friday and Saturday?' The client then rolled off a litany of reasons why it was inappropriate to drink on a Tuesday – work the next day, finance, etc. In elaborating these reasons *A* became more committed to the original goals. He had in fact also stepped into thinking that the drinking he did on the Friday and Saturday were also somehow 'violations' so that he had an overwhelming sense of guilt. The therapist pointed out that in fact on only one of the past eight days had *A* departed from his goals, and that this was much better success in achieving goals than he had experienced in a long time. The client and therapist then worked on developing a set of self-instructions that would provide an antidote to the sort of situation that occurred the previous Tuesday. The slip occurred because *A* had a half-day's leave and felt he must make the most of it – it was the last opportunity he would have for some time to meet a particular friend. He telephoned his friend who suggested they meet in their usual haunt – a pub! *A* felt he couldn't let his friend down, and so with a minimum of guilt met him. As the day wore on his guilt increased and he drank more and more. This scenario is fairly typical of the way clients with addiction problems can make decisions apparently unrelated to their addiction but somehow leading inexorably towards it. In *A*'s case, before making decisions about social contact, he was first to ask himself 'how likely is it, on the basis of past experience, that the contact will lead to unplanned drinking? What are the other options?'

Handling slips

Paradoxically, the more successful a treatment programme has already been with a client, the more traumatic the reaction to any slip that occurs. The client will likely have become deeply attached to a self-image – as a non-addict/non-alcoholic. A slip then constitutes a major threat to his self-identity. The danger is that the slip ushers in such a debilitating sense of guilt that the client seeks to assuage it by taking more of the drug. This phenomenon has been termed the Abstinence Violation Effect (AVE) (Marlatt and Gordon 1985). The AVE arises when the client attributes the slip entirely to himself, because of wide-ranging and permanent deficiency (for example, lack of willpower). Therapeutically the task is for the therapist to teach the client to see a slip as arising out of external factors which he has not yet learnt to master and that it is just a question of refining the technology. Essentially the therapist is conveying 'it wasn't that the task was impossible for you, more that we haven't developed the right tools for the job yet; you can't dig a garden with a spoon no matter how hard you try'. It is useful to liken guilt to anxiety along the lines of:

> A small amount of anxiety is useful – it makes you cautious crossing the road. Too much anxiety means that you could well cause the very thing you are trying to avoid – an accident. Similarly, a small dose of guilt is useful: it brings about reasonable change but too much is no good to yourself or anybody else. The idea is to keep guilt manageable.

Each slip will be an occasion to reconstruct an appropriate set of self-instructions along the lines described earlier. The AVE challenges notions such as 'one drink leads to a drunk' by implying there is no inevitability about this process, and that it very much depends on how the individual chooses to think about the slip that is largely responsible for subsequent behaviour. The continuance of drinking or drug taking is then seen primarily as a decision rather than a physiological inevitability.

Discussion of the AVE with a client, even if there have not already been slips, is important in serving as a preventive measure. Ideally the client's handling of a slip should be role played and a set of self-instructions generated – 'I have slipped, but it doesn't have to become a full-blown relapse. There is no way I am back to square one, look what I have already achieved . . . what can I learn from this situation?' Clients who have not had a slip since the inception of the Programme are, however, often resistant to such discussions, and even more resistant to role plays. The therapist has to capitalise on his established relationship with the client and seek to sell the idea by emphasising that it is an insurance policy 'if it does no good it will do no harm'. Should there be subsequent slips the therapist can refer back to the rehearsal of relapse procedures as a way of reassuring the client that slips were an anticipated part of learning to manage the addiction and that 'the show is still very much on the road'.

Analyses of the situations in which a client slips often indicate attitudes which are approximations to some of the dysfunctional attitudes on the DRAQ mentioned earlier in this chapter. Attitudes may be challenged in a variety of ways:

1. *Validity* – for example, 'You were saying you have nothing to look forward to, but a few weeks ago you mentioned going to the football match which you used to really enjoy'.
2. *Consistency* – 'You don't see *X* as worthless – he may now have recovered from his addiction but he has been an addict a lot longer than yourself. So what makes you worthless?'
3. *Utility* – 'How useful is it to think if you cannot do something well there is little point in doing it at all? Did it actually help you achieve anything in straightening out your flat?'
4. *Authority* – 'Why do you take your current friends' opinion of you as being more likely to be right, than what you think of yourself, or indeed what I think of you? Whose authority do you take, friends of now, or of ten years ago?'
5. *Goal* – 'Are you really that far from achieving the goal you want, is it actually the best goal to pursue, is there another means to the goal?'

These ways of challenging attitudes that maintain addictive behaviours may also be used for challenging attitudes that maintain depression. As depression itself can complicate and serve to maintain an addiction, it is suggested that the reader refer to another text for a detailed description of a cognitive-behavioural approach to depression (Scott 1989).

Managing daily hassles

A client's skill in handling the daily hassles of life can be an important determinant of whether relapse occurs. Clearly how the client handles major life events will also be important, but in the nature of things the latter are more infrequent than the former. The daily hassles can accumulate and produce a pronounced effect in the life of the client. Problem-solving training is ideally suited to teaching clients how to manage the daily hassles. Problem solving begins with as precise a definition of the problem as possible. General areas of dissatisfaction may have been indicated on the social questionnaire completed at initial assessment. The specific nature of the rated dissatisfactions should be probed by the therapist as part of the first step of problem solving. The second stage of problem solving involves the generation of as many alternative solutions as possible without weighing their merits. Third, there is the consideration of the consequences of acting on each of the possible solutions. Fourth, in the light of the various anticipated consequences implementing the solutions which seem best. To return to client *A* – *A*'s alternatives were not to ring the friend/ring the friend and go for a drink/ring the friend and meet to go to an evening football game. With the benefit of hindsight *A* wished he had chosen the last alternative.

The problem-solving approach fits well within the framework of an RP Programme in that the fifth step of the procedure is to test out the utility of the chosen solution and in the light of experience opt for another solution if the first proves impractical. Again, the client is put in the role of a scientist, or more exactly an engineer, about his own experiences, continuing to use that which works, abandoning that which doesn't, searching for and trying out new alternatives.

The problem-solving procedure can be applied to aspects of the client's dissatisfactions with his environment. Dissatisfactions may lower mood and the negative emotional state induced can act as a trigger for drug abuse. Problem solving may be brought to bear, not only in the resolution of impersonal matters such as occupation/daily routine, housing, and finances, but also in the realm of interpersonal conflict. When applied in the interpersonal sphere, problem solving contains a number of key additional features. These include teaching the client first of all to try and understand the conflict from the other person's point of view, to put themselves in the other person's shoes. This enables the client to say something positive before expressing a specific criticism. For example, *B* had become upset about his parents' constant checking of his whereabouts and expressed his concern: 'I know you both stood by through all my drug problem and that it is only out of concern that you check up on me, but please do not ring my friends to check where I am'. In this exchange *B* had paved the way for his parents' acceptance of criticism by saying something positive first, and when the criticism was expressed it was highly specific. The more specific the request, the more able the recipient is to agree or disagree with it, thus enabling the problem-solving process to be taken a stage further. The more 'fuzzy' the requests the more stuck the problem-solving process becomes. If *B* had said, 'I just want you both to change your attitude to me, I am just being watched all the time', the parents would be likely to feel helpless, because the request does not suggest anything definite that they can do. Applied in an interpersonal context, the client is encouraged to be open and a contributor to the widest possible range of solutions to a problem. Those with whom he typically interacts in a conflictual manner are, where possible, encouraged to contribute to the brainstorming. Obviously this process is often much easier if the other party is a spouse or parent rather than say a landlord.

Probably the greatest saboteur of interpersonal cognitive problem solving is the tendency for parties to 'mind read'. In *B*'s case he had been operating on the assumption that his parents didn't really want him to grow up, and therefore had never liked him going out. *B* had concluded that because his parents had protested about a series of friends he had made a year or two ago this meant they wanted to keep him 'the baby of the family' – an arbitrary inference. Part of effective interpersonal problem solving involves the client checking out with the other party that they do hold the attitudes he believes them to hold. It is a useful practice to teach the client to summarise what he thinks the other party has said, check it out in a non-threatening way, before making his reply. For occasions on which the client feels his anger is rising, it is useful to have him visualise a set of traffic lights. The lights are on red shouting STOP! As they move to amber he instructs himself to 'play it cool, think how I can play this to my best advantage, what are the alternatives'. Having paused to reflect on the alternatives the client selects one. As the lights change to green he visualises himself slowly moving off in the direction of the chosen solution. Most solutions arrived at by the client in dialogue with other parties will likely involve mutuality and compromise and are capable of being expressed in a specific manner. In *B*'s case, for his part he agreed that he would be home by 11.30 p.m. each evening whilst his parents agreed not to telephone his friends. Essentially in interpersonal cognitive problem solving the client is being taught how to be assertive – balancing his own needs against those of others. This does not, however, mean that the result of each attempt at problem solving has to be a compromise, but simply that overall there is a concern to balance needs.

The social pressures to abuse drugs or drink call for specific assertive responses in relation to these substances. Foy *et al.* (1976) developed a technique called 'refusal training' for such instances. The components of a refusal response are:

1. Direct eye contact.
2. Serious and expressive voice tone.
3. An attempt to change the subject of the conversation.
4. Offering an alternative. For example, a person with a drink problem might say, 'No thanks I'll try a . . . (non-alcoholic beer).'
5. Requesting the pusher not to ask again.

The refusal response should be practised via role plays in the session and the client should also be asked to practise the scenes in imagination for homework.

The pursuit of life goals

A Relapse Prevention Programme obviously has as one of its targets a modification of the client's addictive behaviour. But it was suggested at the start of the chapter that it is only adopted and maintained by clients in a context in which other more meaningful goals are possible. The implications of this are that, should life goals disappear off the client's horizon during the course of a programme, the client is likely to default. It follows that an important element of an RP Programme is a specification of life goals to be pursued and the detailing of steps along the way to their realisation. If multiple goals are delineated this allows the client some sense of achievement, even if the roadblocks to the pursuit of a particular goal are proving insuperable. The therapist can help the client gauge how near he is to the realisation of goals and perhaps enlarge the range of means to pursue various goals. The range of possible client actions is more limited in some social contexts than others. Life-style modification may be a very meaningful concept for some addicted persons, but for many in the inner cities of Britain there are very real limitations to the range of options therapists and clients can create. This clearly raises economic and political issues beyond the scope of this chapter.

The life goals pursued may be of two types – achievement or relationship orientated, depending on the personality of the client, or a mix of both, if the client so wishes. Ambitions the client nursed before the addictive behaviour can be a useful starting point in discussing possible life goals. Some clients seem never to have had any ambitions of any sort. This could be a simple statement of fact, no possibilities had ever suggested themselves, or it could be that the client eradicated thoughts of ambition for fear of the consequences of failing to realise the ambition. If it is the latter, the 'catastrophic' interpretation of failure experience would need challenging using cognitive techniques (see Scott 1989). Standard social skills programmes may be a useful adjunct to an RP Programme for clients deficient in such skills, but with life goals that are primarily relationship orientated. Most social skills packages tend to concentrate on the skills necessary to initiate contact with people rather than those necessary to maintain a relationship. The integration of the interpersonal cognitive problem-solving strategies, described earlier, into social skills programmes, helps to achieve a balance between initiation and maintenance skills. Scott (1989) has developed a programme giving equal emphasis to skills of initiation and maintenance.

Maintaining vigilance

The RPP rests on quite different principles to the disease or medical model of treatment as the completer on an RP Programme cannot regard themselves as 'cured'. The completer, like someone who has learnt to drive a car and passed his driving test, is only safe in so far as he or she continues to practise the skills learnt. With the passage of time details of lessons are often forgotten. In order to consolidate the learning that has taken place in the core, RPP booster sessions at monthly intervals are recommended. These sessions are invaluable in that the client has by this time a wealth of experience of practising a non-addictive life-style, and particular vulnerabilities will be the more readily apparent. Material perhaps mentioned but not given any prominence at an earlier session may be re-examined and its relevance in addressing demonstrated vulnerabilities underlined. Clients tend, after the core programme, to want to push to the background any literature or pro formas used because they serve as a reminder of a painful period of their life. Having clients develop and continue to utilise their own 'Bible' is most useful. In the core programme client *C* completed a record about occasions he became upset, recording what happened, how he felt, what it sounded 'as if' he was saying to himself in the situation, and finally the rational responses. Much of his upset had to do with feelings of loneliness which he was able to come to terms with using the thought records. However, on seeing *C* for a three-month booster session, he was again feeling isolated but had completely 'forgotten' about using the thought records. After this booster session *C* recommenced the thought records and thus removed the sense of self-blame for being lonely, enabling him to plan a new social life.

References

Corney, R.H. and Clare, A.W. (1985) 'The construction development and testing of a self-report questionnaire to identify social problems', *Psychological Medicine*, 15: 637–49.

Cummings, C., Gordon, J.R., and Marlatt, G.A. (1980) 'Relapse: prevention and prediction', in W.R. Miller (ed.) *The Addictive Behaviours*, Oxford: Pergamon Press.

Foy, D.W., Miller, P.M., Eisler, R.M., and O'Toole, D.H. (1976) 'Social skills training to teach alcoholics to refuse drinks effectively', *Journal of Alcohol Studies*, 37: 1340–5.

Litman, G.K., Stapleton, J., Openheim, A.N., Peleg, M., and Jackson, P. (1983) 'Situations related to alcoholism relapse', *British Journal of*

Addiction, 78: 381–9.
Marlatt, G.A. and Gordon, J.R. (1985) *Relapse Prevention*, New York: Guilford Press.
Prochaska, J.O. and DiClemente, C.C. (1982) 'Transtheoretical therapy: toward a more integrative model of change', *Psychotherapy: Theory, Research and Practice*, 19: 276–88.
Scott, M.J. (1989) *A Cognitive-Behavioural Approach to Clients' Problems*, London: Routledge.

Chapter Six

Medical treatment for problem drug takers

Nas Choudry

Introduction

Medical treatment is an important component of comprehensive services for problem drug takers. The possibility of prescribing drugs such as methadone attracts problem opiate takers into contact with services, thus providing opportunities for the social and psychological interventions described in other chapters. Having a clear understanding of current medical practices and of recent developments in this area enables non-prescribing drug workers to co-operate most effectively with medical practitioners whether they be general practitioners or psychiatrists. This chapter focuses solely on medical treatments in order to present current standards of good practice particularly related to detoxification. It recognises the wider issues of prescribing policies (discussed by Wilks in Chapter 9) but confines itself to practical clinical issues.

Drug-dependence clinics need to develop full assessment procedures and be very familiar with the changing local drug scenes so that needs can be identified early and met. Knowledge of other local services provided by both statutory and voluntary bodies is essential to avoid duplication of services and to link the facilities available. If possible the size and nature of the local drug problem should be ascertained. Surveys in East Dorset have been used to involve probation and social services and to emphasise the important needs of comprehensive school children (Pritchard *et al.* 1985, 1986).

On referral

Immediately on referral it is important to check with the Home Office Drugs Branch to see if the patient has been notified to them and if any treatment, particularly the prescribing of controlled drugs, is currently available to them. This simple step will go some way to preventing the problems of dual prescribing and will give some indication of the patient's previous involvement with services. If at all possible, prior to attendance at the clinic, contact can be made via the Community Drug Team (CDT) so that at least initial problems can begin to be identified.

On attendance

If the appointment has been made following a referral from a general practitioner, there is always the possibility that the patient may not turn up at the clinic: this is less likely in those with problems with opiates. A full systematic history needs to be obtained and a fixed format can be used to ensure complete and accurate information on all aspects of the individual's functioning. If the referral has not come directly from a general practitioner a full clinical examination should be advised to look at least for puncture marks, bearing in mind the common sites of injection, that is, antecubital fossae, arms, wrists, hands, ankles, feet, groin, armpits, shoulders, breasts, and at times the neck, confirming any history of abuse by mainlining (injection). Further confirmation of the consumption of the drug is important and can be carried out by urinary analysis using one of the systems which can give almost immediate results, for example, the EMIT-ST urinary scan machine. This can be adapted for use in the clinic and can check the urine for opiates, methadone, amphetamines, cocaine, barbiturates, benzodiazepines, and others if so wished. This is an important step and it would be difficult to run a prescribing clinic without this facility. It is also important because there can be discrepancies between the drugs that the individuals believe themselves to have taken and those that are in their system. That is, they may be inadvertently abusing several drugs because of adulteration of 'street' supplies with cheaper alternatives (Choudry and Doe 1986).

The variety of drugs found in the urine of fifty consecutive heroin addicts attending the clinic in East Dorset in 1986 is displayed in Table 6.1. Amphetamines and barbiturates were found to be the drugs which were most often taken inadvertently. Polydrug abuse remains a problem, as shown in Table 6.2. This lists all of the drugs identified in the urine of fifty-two patients on their first attendance at the clinic in East Dorset. Only in 54 per cent of cases was just one drug present: the rest had two or more.

Once the dependency and the drug has been confirmed, the various options available can be discussed and offered to the patient.

Table 6.1 Nature of drugs (known and inadvertent) detected in the urine of fifty heroin addicts in 1986

	Opiates	*Methadone*	*Amphetamines*	*Barbiturates*	*Cocaine*	*Benzo-diazepines*
Known	50 (100%)	9 (18%)	11 (22%)	2 (4%)	2 (4%)	7 (14%)
Inadvertent	0	0	8 (16%)	8 (16%)	0	3 (6%)

Source: Choudry 1986

Table 6.2 Drugs present in the urine of fifty-two heroin addicts on their first attendance at the East Dorset Clinic in 1986

Numbers of drugs present in each patient	1	2	3	4	
Number of patients with this number of drugs present	28 (54%)	16 (31%)	7 (13%)	1 (2%)	
Frequencies of types of drugs					*Drug totals (%)*
Opiates	12	13	7	1	33 (39)
Methadone	6	5	5	1	17 (20)
Cocaine	1	1	1	0	3 (3)
Barbiturates	0	1	2	1	4 (5)
Benzodiazepines	3	6	3	1	13 (15)
Amphetamines	6	6	3	0	15 (18)

Note: Only twenty-eight patients had just one drug present.
Source: Choudry 1986

Options available for opiate abusers

Detoxification

Withdrawal without medical cover is sometimes possible with the support of voluntary organisations, family, or friends. It is usually not a preferred option and can be difficult to manage from the carers' point of view. It is important, however, to appreciate that 'cold turkey' is possible in highly motivated individuals and with the right support. A non-prescribing programme for narcotic users exists in Sheffield and this appears to have the support of a number of agencies and could well be a satisfactory option for certain districts who are setting up services (Liappas *et al.* 1987).

In-patient detoxification

This can be carried out either in an acute medical or psychiatric ward, or in a special drug-dependency in-patient unit. The advantages of the latter will include the initiation of a rehabilitation programme particularly geared towards the problems of addictions. However, some patients may well prefer a straightforward detoxification and then work in the community supported by other services, for example, from the Community Drug Team. There are several options for the in-patient detoxification of opiate dependents. These include:

1. Detoxification with tranquillisers, and avoiding the use of controlled drugs. This method is not very readily chosen and can be problematic in holding the patient in therapy. It can be useful for those who have been partly withdrawn as out-patients and who wish to come into hospital for the last period of detoxification. The use of thioridazine or chlorpromazine can be considered along with benzodiazepines in the short term.
2. Methadone reducing-dose regimes geared for the needs of the patient can be initiated and the dosages titrated according to withdrawal effects, and is a much more controlled method of detoxification. The usual precautions are necessary with regard to the taking of drugs 'smuggled' into the ward environment and can produce problems in management. Recent work confirms the importance of the influence of psychological factors on the opiate withdrawal syndrome. Withdrawal symptoms can be protracted and may not return to normal until about twenty days after the end of the withdrawal regime, and their severity may not be dose related (Gossop, Bradley, and Phillips 1987). It is thus crucial to add psychological support to detoxification programmes using methadone (Phillips, Gossop, and Bradley, 1986).
3. Clonidine detoxification: clonidine, an alpha-2 adrenergic agonist used in the treatment of migraine and hypertension in medical practice, has proved to be useful in the treatment of opiate dependents. Given orally the dosages can be reduced over about a two-week period, and in-patient status allows the sedative and hypotensive side effects to be carefully monitored and dosages adjusted as necessary. It appears to be better tolerated by patients detoxified immediately from illicit opiates and can prove difficult to use in patients stabilised on high doses of methadone, possibly over 20 mg daily. It is a non-opiate and thus all the problems related to prescribing a controlled drug can be avoided.

Out-patient withdrawal

Without opiate substitutes

With the use of major tranquillisers, for example, thioridazine, chlorpromazine, or perphenazine, it is possible to withdraw opiate dependents who are highly motivated. The dosages can be titrated to the degree of clinical symptoms and this can be monitored with 'key carers' through an out-patient clinic. The use of hypnotics should be restricted to short-term use due to their own dependency problems, but they can be a useful addition, particularly in the early phases of the treatment programme.

With opiates

Drug clinics, when established in the mid to late 1960s, used diamorphine ampoules, and it is theoretically possible to prescribe this on a reducing dose basis, but it is difficult to administer and supervise. A special licence is needed from the Home Office for a practitioner to prescribe diamorphine to opiate dependents. The use of codeine phosphate tablets is sometimes possible in the withdrawal of patients who are particularly dependent on codeine. Other opioids, for example dipipanone (particularly in combination with cyclizine and marketed under the trade name, Diconal), dextromoramide, and buprenorphine, have been used, but with accompanying difficulties of ongoing abuse, particularly the intravenous injection of crushed tablets. In response to the resulting fatalities dipipanone was placed on the restricted list in 1985. It is important to be aware of the dangers of crushing and injecting tablets specifically designed to be taken orally, and in this aspect suspensions and mixtures may be advisable.

With opiate substitutes

The most commonly used opiate substitute is methadone which has been available since the Second World War. It is a potent analgesic with a long half life, and thus once substituted for diamorphine can be reduced over a variable period of time. It is available in ampoules (for injection), tablets, linctus (2 mg in 5 ml), and mixture (1 mg in 1 ml). The use of ampoules and tablets is to be discouraged and many centres now are using the methadone mixture. This can be prescribed by any medical practitioner and requires no central licence. The use of ampoules and tablets has led to abuse, and these preparations have more of a black market value than the mixture. The amount of mixture used will depend on the amount of street heroin consumed and its potency, but it is usual to start at a safe dosage of between 30 and 50 mg daily for opiate dependents consuming half to one gramme of street heroin per day either by smoking (chasing) or by injection (mainlining). The contract of withdrawal time can be negotiated with the patient and can vary depending on the age, maturity, motivation, support, and the length and severity of the addiction. Good working relationships with the local hospital and retail pharmacists are desirable so that any abuse can be identified early and corrected. Due to the high sugar content of the preparations it is wise to advise the patients to use a straw when drinking the mixture to minimise the risk of dental decay, particularly when the prescription is high and for a lengthy period of time. It is important to implement the prescribing with intensive and consistent support from a Community Drug Team or other services so as to ensure ongoing motivation and crisis intervention. It is often necessary to renegotiate the contracts of withdrawal and it should be possible, with urine analysis, preferably using on-the-spot check systems, for example, the EMIT system, to ensure that the terms of the contract are adhered to, or at least to keep the pressure on the patient to engineer continuing motivation. The use of methadone mixture during pregnancy is relatively safe, at least safer than ongoing abuse of street heroin, and it is to be remembered that small proportions of it do filter through to the developing foetus and also into breast milk. The management of the pregnant problem drug taker is an important issue, and every care and precaution should be taken (Riley, 1987).

With other preparations

Clonidine. This drug is now well established on the withdrawal of opiate addiction. However, due to its ability to produce postural hypotension and sedation, its use is often limited to in-patients. It is being used for out-patients in some centres but it is necessary to ensure daily contact with the patients so any side effects, particularly low blood pressure, can be monitored and this may be possible for example through the Community Psychiatric Nurse (CPN) of a Community Drugs Team. Further work is needed in its use for out-patients before it can be generally recommended.

Naltrexone. The use of naltrexone is established in some centres, particularly in the United States, and needs to be fully evaluated. Naltrexone was first synthesised in 1965 by Bloomberg, and it was found to be an orally effective, long-acting, good narcotic antagonist. It is thought to be useful for opiate dependents who have been detoxified and who have a high risk of relapse. In opiate dependents prior to complete detoxification it will trigger off acute withdrawal symptoms and hence needs the full co-operation of a motivated patient. It will actually block the opiate receptors so that the intake of an opiate following naltrexone treatment will have no clinical effect, eliminating the 'buzz' that is so important in the drug taking. There is some work to suggest that clonidine detoxification followed by naltrexone used on a regular basis may prove to be a useful therapy for some motivated patients. Out-patient treatment will have to be carefully monitored since the administration of this substance to dependent individuals will trigger off acute withdrawal. There is some evidence that the use of naltrexone in combination with psychological treatment can be beneficial in some patients. In the UK Brewer has had some experience with this preparation and claims, following a review of seventy patients, that in combination with clonidine and diazepam, naltrexone permits safe, rapid and acceptable detoxification with a drop-out rate of less than 2 per cent (Brewer 1987). He argues that supervised naltrexone is a very useful addition to the management of several aspects of opiate abuse. Naltrexone has only been available for prescription by medical practitioners in the UK since the summer of 1988 and its full potential can now be evaluated.

Medical treatment of the stimulant dependent

The main drugs in this group include amphetamines and cocaine, and to a lesser extent drugs with stimulant properties, for example, Tenuate, Dospan, and some nasal decongestants. Dependence on amphetamines and cocaine can be a very difficult state to treat medically since there are no drugs available which will block the 'highs' induced by them. The withdrawal effects of any drugs, on the whole, are exactly the opposite of their pharmacological effects so the stimulant-dependent individual will normally 'sleep off' the drugs in the first 48 to 72 hours and then be left with strong psychological cravings and, with the lethargy and weakness experienced, the need for further intake is great. Tricyclic antidepressants, especially desipramine given in doses as required, can play a part in minimising these cravings, and combined with intensive support of a psychological nature they can be helpful. An amphetamine-induced depression with some biological features can also be controlled by the use of the tricyclics, and should be considered since there is a real threat to reabuse in spite of intensive support. The benzodiazepines and hypnotics should be used with caution and should not continue for any lengthy period of time due to their own potential for dependence. Amphetamine-induced psychosis which has strong paranoid qualities, and has many of the features of state similar to paranoid schizophrenia, can follow heavy use of amphetamines over a short period of time, and will settle in two to three weeks, and can be helped by the use of the major neuroleptics as can continuing paranoid symptoms. Amphetamines can trigger off episodes of paranoid schizophrenia in vulnerable individuals who tend to have a preference for amphetamines as a drug of abuse. Such persons are also at risk to some street heroin which is laced with significant amounts of amphetamines, enough, sometimes, to trigger off paranoid states. Cocaine dependency can be severe and difficult to treat: with prices dropping, suggesting more availability, it is becoming a problem to the drug services. The tactile hallucinations, the so called 'cocaine bug', is a classical effect following the abuse of this drug and may need major neuroleptics in its management. Management of the cocaine dependent needs a whole range of support mechanisms ranging from family to the Community Drugs Team to minimise the craving which can lead to reabuse.

Medical treatment of the sedative dependents

The main drugs in this section are the barbiturates which can be considered as 'dry drink', and the withdrawal effects are very similar to the withdrawal from alcohol. Full-blown delirium tremens and epileptic fits can be observed and will need, usually, in-patient management and close supervision and sedation.

The abuse of pure barbiturates is not common and they are usually taken advertently or inadvertently with street heroin, and can complicate the presentation in the withdrawal stages. The shorter-acting barbiturates (for example, amylobarbitone), due to their immediate 'buzz', are more prone to abuse than the longer-acting phenobarbitone, used in the treatment of epilepsy, and crushed tablets have been used to lace the street heroin thus giving it bite and bulk. There exists a core of elderly dependents who have had prescriptions for barbiturate hypnotics for very many years, and it is interesting that many of them have remained on the same dosages for this period of time. Recent removals by pharmaceutical companies of some of these barbiturate preparations, for example, nembutal, from general use, have caused difficulties for some of these patients who have had problems in converting to other preparations, and provides an opportunity to take them off the barbiturate hypnotics.

Medical treatment of benzodiazepine dependents

A major problem exists with dependency on the benzodiazepines highlighted by the media over the last few years. It is clear that all of the present benzodiazepines have the capability of producing a dependency state, some more than others, for example, lorazepam more than clorazepate. The medical treatment has to take into account the slow reduction regime with controlled prescriptions coupled with group or individual support through Tranx groups or through a Community Drug Team. The somatic symptoms during withdrawal can be intense and varied and the presentation can be complicated by hyperventilation and its sequelae. Anxiety management, relaxation training, and rebreathing can all be seen as part of the overall management of these patients.

The abuse of benzodiazepine hypnotics (for example, Temazepam, Triazolam) by injection of the crushed tablets is of increasing concern, and these drugs can be used to lace supplies of street heroin and consequently they have a black market value. General prescribing habits need to be maintained to ensure some control of the abuse.

Medical management of the abuse of hallucinogenics

Hallucinogens, for example, LSD and magic mushrooms, have always been in the background of the drug culture. The management in the acute stages may need hospitalisation and treatment with neuroleptics and settles quickly. There is no place for any medication after this unless specific psychiatric symptoms have been detected which may respond to anxiolytics, antidepressants or major neuroleptics. A full support mechanism through a number of channels needs to be set up around the individual.

Medical treatment of solvent abuse

Acute medical emergencies are a feature of this substance abuse with sometimes fatal results, and a wide variety of solvent-based products can be used. Management of these acute stages may include neuroleptics to control the agitation and toxic state which will settle over a few hours. No specific medical management is necessary after this, and a full network of support systems needs to be established. Education of the medical complications is crucial in any preventative programme and there needs to be community involvement in its management (Barnes 1979; Sourindhrin and Baird 1984).

Medical treatment of cannabis abuse

The use of cannabis is widespread and in all parts of society in long term and heavy use has been thought to cause various organic changes which have never been fully evaluated. In vulnerable individuals a cannabis induced psychosis can occur which can be long lasting and difficult to treat even in spite of intensive pharmacological treatment. It is very much an established behaviour in the drug culture and being illegal it is currently found where other illegal drugs are also found, thus making available these other drugs to vulnerable individuals who may only be after cannabis.

References

Barnes, G.E. (1979) 'Solvent abuse: a review', *International Journal of Addiction*, 14: 1–26.

Brewer, C. (1987) 'Naltrexone in the management of opiate abuse: experiences with rapid withdrawal and the prevention and detection of relapse. A review of 70 cases', *British Journal of Addiction*, 82: 1369.

Choudry, N. (1986) *A district looks at its drug problems*. Unpublished report, East Dorset Health Authority.

Choudry, N. and Doe, J. (1986) 'Inadvertent abuse of amphetamines in street heroin', *The Lancet*, 4 October, 8510: 817.

Gossop, M., Bradley, B., and Phillips, G. (1987) 'An investigation of withdrawal symptoms shown by opiate addicts during and subsequent to a twenty-one day inpatient methadone detoxification procedure', *Addictive Behaviours*, 12: 1–6.

Liappas, J.A., Jenner, F.A., Vlissides, D.N., and Vicente, B. (1987) 'Thoughts on the Sheffield non-prescribing programme for narcotic users', *British Journal of Addiction*, 82: 999–1006.

Phillips, G.T., Gossop, M., and Bradley, B. (1986) 'The influence of psychological factors on the opiate withdrawal syndrome', *British Journal of Psychiatry*, 149: 235–8.

Pritchard, C., Fielding, M., Choudry, N., Cox, M., and Swan, C. (1985) 'Drug and solvent abuse in the caseload of probation and social services departments: a balanced approach', *Community Care*, 570: 25–7.

Pritchard, C., Fielding, M., Choudry, N., Cox, M., and Diamond, I. (1986) 'Incidence of drug and solvent abuse in normal fourth and fifth year comprehensive school children. Some sociobehavioural characteristics', *British Journal of Social Work*, 16: 341–51.

Riley, D. (1987) 'Management of the pregnant drug addict', *Bulletin of the Royal College of Psychiatrists*, 11: 12–28.

Sourindhrin, I. and Baird, J.A. (1984) 'Management of solvent misuse: A Glasgow community approach', *British Journal of Addiction*, 79: 227–32.

Chapter Seven

Managing benzodiazepine withdrawal

Moira Hamlin and Diane Hammersley

Introduction

Why manage tranquilliser withdrawal?

Recent years have seen an increase in media attention to the problems of dependence on tranquillisers, much of it focusing on the disabling physical and psychological side effects. Many tranquilliser users and ex-users have written or spoken about their difficulties and distress in trying to withdraw from these drugs. Many have described feelings of guilt at the discovery of their own 'addiction' or anger that they had become dependent involuntarily.

The search for information and sound advice has led many to start or join self-help groups or to seek advice from their general practitioners or drug-counselling agencies, both statutory and voluntary. The public has already received the message that tranquillisers are not the once-hoped-for safe alternative to barbiturates, but have many adverse side effects as well as a dependence potential. New guidelines on prescribing have been issued, limiting the use of tranquillisers to a maximum of four weeks and then only as a treatment of last resort (Committee on the Safety of Medicines 1988; Royal College of Psychiatrists 1988).

It is for those already dependent on tranquillisers, for a few weeks or over twenty-five years, that attention is now being directed towards finding a safe effective way to help those who wish to withdraw. Increasingly it is being recognised that tranquillisers were only ever of use as a temporary measure of symptomatic relief (Committee on the Review of Medicines 1980). Those who withdraw from them may also require further help to deal with psychosocial problems, of which anxiety was an indication.

It is understandable that people dependent on tranquillisers should feel that the best thing to do is to stop taking them immediately. Indeed some have been advised to do so, especially when on very low doses, until it became evident that withdrawal even from very low doses has its own particular difficulty.

People have looked to alternative medicine, herbal remedies, homoeopathy, acupuncture and hypnotherapy, and other therapies as alternatives to tranquillisers to help them withdraw. These may be valid and useful in their way but they are not all that is required. Switching to an alternative therapy fails to pay proper attention to physical dependence. A pharmacological understanding of tranquilliser withdrawal is also required.

A second approach has been to see withdrawal as largely a pharmacological problem. The search for drugs of substitution, or to minimise the withdrawal syndrome, or even the availability of a 'non-addictive' alternative have failed to recognise the psychological aspects. Measuring how quickly the tranquillisers can be eliminated from the body and scheduling people to reduce accordingly does not allow time to make the necessary adjustments as they proceed. This can leave people bewildered, frightened and hopeless. Effects of too rapid withdrawal or sudden cessation of medication may mean, among other things, that the person becomes severely agoraphobic, polyphobic, obsessional, requires in-patient treatment, or has long periods off work while they restore the psychological balance of their lives.

Clearly what is sought is an integrated approach to tranquilliser withdrawal which pays proper attention to both physical and psychological aspects. It is crucial that tranquillisers are not seen as the same as any other drug which has a dependence potential. In general, established techniques which may be safe and effective for withdrawal from other substances may not always be appropriate for this group of drugs. The withdrawal may take much longer than most people expect. Unrealistic expectations can be worrying and frustrating for both the client, the helping agency, and the general practitioner.

We have found that people who have withdrawn from tranquillisers may report that they are still experiencing the withdrawal syndrome months or even years after they have stopped taking tranquillisers. It is both puzzling and frustrating when they continue to request help from their doctors and others for unspecific symptoms which appear to resist treatment!

This chapter considers (a) different types of individual and group treatment programmes, (b) assessment and clinical decision-making, (c) running withdrawal groups, and (d) what the worker needs to know about tranquillisers and withdrawing from them. Further details of this approach to tranquilliser withdrawal, group leaders' notes and copies of the session handouts are included in the

WITHDRAW Teaching Pack currently being prepared for publication. Throughout, the client is referred to as 'she' as the majority of tranquilliser clients are women. The worker is referred to as 'he' for balance; it may be understood that in both cases men and women are included.

An integrated approach

The advantage of an integrated approach is that it deals with all aspects of withdrawal from the start. It must clearly be better practice to consider the frequently described forms of agoraphobia, for example, in conjunction with withdrawal, rather than leaving the client drug free but afraid to leave the home alone. In withdrawing from tranquillisers the client has an implicit hope that the quality of life will improve.

Several studies have begun to consider what might be needed psychologically in addition to controlled withdrawal from tranquillisers. These are described in more detail and reviewed elsewhere (Hamlin 1988). Non-medical interventions tried have included sympathetic listening and reassurance, anxiety management including relaxation training and positive thinking, and behaviour therapy. All these non-medical treatments may be helpful psychologically but for whom? Tranquilliser users are not a homogeneous group. Those who have other difficulties in addition to tranquilliser dependence may need a more therapeutic intervention and demand more skilled help. The task is clearly to look for interventions appropriate for tranquilliser withdrawal which can be shown to work and which meet the needs of a wide variety of users.

The WITHDRAW Project

The WITHDRAW Project was established to offer a clinical psychological service to people who wanted to withdraw from tranquillisers. It is unique in that it has a research study running parallel with it which allows for the research findings to influence the development of the clinical service and for clinical impressions to be investigated by research. It aims to identify those people who may successfully withdraw from tranquillisers, to assess the severity of the psychological problems before and after treatment, and to evaluate the WITHDRAW three-tier model of intervention.

The first tier consists mostly of information, the second is a short-term group approach run by a psychologist or counsellor, and the third tier is a longer-term group offering a more in-depth therapeutic intervention. A fundamental aim is to go beyond tranquilliser withdrawal, which is relatively easy, to teach alternative coping strategies, so that people maintain the withdrawal, and stay off tranquillisers.

Areas which the group approach includes are depression, anxiety, low self-esteem, and isolation – whether these were problems before or while taking tranquillisers, or during withdrawal. Here the aim is to change the tacit acceptance of medication as a valid solution to social or psychological difficulties. Psychological methods have more potential than medication for developing effective coping strategies both for withdrawal and life stress.

Treatment options

Choice of treatment – individual or group

If an individual programme is considered for clients it is important to weigh up the advantages and disadvantages of this option against those of a group approach:

1. The client may have the undivided attention and skills of the worker but will lose the opportunity to discover that she is not the only person with the problem. Recognition of this does much to relieve the shame and guilt associated with drugs or mental disorders.
2. Individual treatment offers the opportunity to set specific mutually agreed goals and ways of achieving them. The treatment can be 'tailor made' to the individual client but it limits the client who may not be aware of, or open to, other possibilities for change. However, clients may experience unexpected gains from taking part in a group where part of the time is spent on 'other people's problems and difficulties'. This also enables the client to learn to handle her own difficulties in a new way by developing strategies for other members of the group.
3. The client in individual treatment is able to look at her use of tablets in an active way, exploring positive new patterns and letting go negative ones in relation to the worker. In a group each client is also able to receive encouragement, support, and a positive view of herself from the other members of the group as well as the worker.
4. Individual sessions may be requested to fit in with family commitments, employment, shift-work, or because of other difficulties such as agoraphobia, or a disinclination to listen to

other people's problems. In practice, reasons such as these, though plausible, often mask other difficulties, such as an unwillingness on the part of the client to pay sufficient attention to her own needs or avoidance of difficult tasks such as asking for time off work or telling other people about the problem. Fear of being swamped by other people's problems may indicate a previous unsatisfactory group experience which needs to be explored, and decisions for individual treatment because of agoraphobia may ignore the fact that taking part in a group could be part of the therapy.

5. Individual treatment can sometimes start immediately, and this seems an attractive option which avoids the time-consuming problems associated with getting together a group of eight to ten people in one place at one time. Group work seems cost-effective but is not as time-saving as is often imagined. However, there are advantages in delaying treatment since the very fact that people can drop out before the treatment programme is a test of the client's motivation. A waiting period allows the client time to consider the changes she is going to make and prepare for them. It may allow the client to distance herself from the worker if she has fears about becoming too dependent on the worker.
6. Clients often express an initial reluctance to join a group and it would be easy for the worker to then opt for individual treatment. In our experience, once clients have joined a group, they gain much benefit from other members. By the end of treatment, many report being appreciative of having been part of a group.

The choice of individual treatment

1. The first option for treatment is one of information and advice only. For some clients who prefer to withdraw on their own, advice, written material, and support either through telephone counselling or one to two appointments may be all they require. Clients who may benefit from this level of treatment may (a) not have been taking tranquillisers for very long, (b) have received other help from elsewhere, or (c) have almost completed withdrawal.
2. Sometimes individual treatment may be used in conjunction with a short group approach either before or after the group withdrawal course. It seems appropriate to offer one to two individual sessions (not in the client's home but preferably at the place where the group will be held) before the course starts for

clients who are agoraphobic, if that treatment option is on offer. Similarly a chaotic user may need an individual session to help stabilise tablet use before the group starts.

3. A third possibility may be to offer one or two individual sessions following the course to discuss issues which have arisen for the client as a result of her withdrawal from tranquillisers. It may also be helpful for clients who are looking for their next step to have a chance to discuss with the worker additional treatment or a referral elsewhere.
4. The worker might also consider offering a client an individual session if something occurs during the course which needs to be dealt with privately. However, in order to preserve the group process, it would be important to 'feed' this back to the group later in order not to encourage competition and secrets.

The short-term group

1. If information/advice alone is insufficient, the second option for treatment is a short-term group led by a trained group worker. The aim is not only to help people stop taking tranquillisers, but also to learn alternative coping strategies. A significant proportion of clients in this category are those who have attempted to stop several times and may have had periods of abstinence. They seem to have developed strategies for reducing the tablets, but the real problem for them is *maintenance* – staying off tranquillisers. It is important to recognise that many groups are run with the express purpose of withdrawing from tranquillisers. This seems short-sighted as there is every indication that during future stress relapse will occur unless new coping strategies have been well learned.
2. A group ideally consists of eight to twelve clients led by a psychologist or counsellor meeting for one and a half hours weekly. The course lasts for eight sessions with the last two sessions at fortnightly intervals and is followed by a booster session three months after the last session. The group is a closed one with clients asked to commit themselves to attending every session and clients are rarely accepted if they miss more than the first session. This is necessary with a short-term group in order to avoid having to 're-start' when a new member joins. Those who are ill at the start of the course, or are unable to attend, may be offered places in a later group but rarely with a different worker.
3. Although withdrawal from tranquillisers is the main aim of people attending groups, the approach adopted is to focus on the

issues underlying and maintaining tranquilliser use. Each session deals with a separate topic, and by the end of the course clients will have had the opportunity to acquire new skills, attitudes, and beliefs. This new learning will help them to continue withdrawing from tranquillisers and resist relapse in the future. Guidelines and advice on how to withdraw are offered, but the pace of this process is determined by the client. Stopping taking tranquillisers may be accomplished quite quickly or take up to a year or more in some cases.

The long-term group

1. The third option of a longer-term group is reserved for those who need more than the first two levels. Clients may have all the facts and information needed on how to withdraw; may understand what they can do instead of taking tranquillisers; they may even have the skills, and yet still fail to give up tranquillisers. More intensive therapy is needed to look at the fundamental issues which may be maintaining tranquilliser use.
2. The kinds of problems which clients in this category might have include unresolved bereavements, chronic agoraphobia, or recurrent relationship difficulties. In practice, clients with one or more of these difficulties are sometimes accepted into a short-term group because, although it may not be all they need, it is all that is available. The group may be at least the start of therapy for them, and the worker needs to be clear about setting appropriate goals and hoping for a realistic outcome.
3. Clients who would benefit very little from a short-term group, and who would differ sufficiently to make them difficult to integrate, are likely to require a long-term group. These clients would fulfil at least four of the following criteria:

   (a) Previous use of illegal drugs; former problem drinkers; excessive and chaotic use of tranquillisers; history of overdosing.
   (b) Unresolved bereavements, multiple bereavements or other major losses with pathological reactions.
   (c) Recurrent relationship difficulties – socially withdrawn, those living alone with few contacts.
   (d) Poor attachment to parents in early childhood (for example, long separations at an early age, physical or emotional abuse).
   (e) Evidence of violence, sexual abuse, or attempted suicide.
   (f) History of psychiatric interventions, including anti-psychotic drugs or ECT.

In these cases there is often an interaction between the tranquillisers and the other psychological problems, and both aspects must be addressed in therapy. A long-term group may consist of fewer clients and last for at least six months in two blocks of ten weeks with a break in the middle. We were constrained in our long-term group because of the end of the Project. Long term is usually one to two years.

Maintenance and support

Two categories of client who may need help are those who:

(a) have attended a short-term or long-term WITHDRAW group and are continuing to withdraw from tranquillisers and make the appropriate changes in their lives;
(b) have withdrawn from tranquillisers either on their own using telephone advice or books, or with advice from their general practitioner.

Both groups of clients may request further support but usually know how to come off tranquillisers. For the first group who are continuing with a process already begun, the need is for continued support and the opportunity to seek help with difficulties as they arise.

The second group are likely to have been unaware at the beginning that anything other than tablet reduction was involved. They now face the problem of maintaining themselves off tranquillisers without knowing what to do instead of taking tablets, without new learning and new skills. Underlying psychological difficulties may still persist and characteristically they lack insight into themselves and their former dependence, and are often impatient or angry because the outcome of withdrawal has not met their expectations.

However, since both groups have a common element in needing to continue looking at their other difficulties while learning and practising new skills for living a drug-free life, a less intensive group may be held less frequently. One opportunity for further support which does not encourage dependence on the worker is an open group, with clients choosing to attend on a sessional basis, and where the relationship with the worker is more distanced. One session of one and a half hours per month might cover such topics as relaxation, assertiveness, bereavement, and dealing with difficult feelings.

The content of the maintenance group sessions may consist of an opportunity to seek further help or support with reducing or staying off. Here the worker may shift the emphasis to exercises which use the learning of other group members. Clients develop their own coping strategies and self-confidence through listening to and supporting others. A second part of the session may concentrate on learning new skills for living – important in living a drug-free life. Topics could include relaxation, assertiveness, coping with criticism, dealing with anger, bereavement and loss, asking for what you want, and fair fighting. Programmes for each season covering up to six months are mailed to people who have been through WITHDRAW groups. Clients ring and book a place on a sessional basis.

The maintenance group seems to be an effective way to incorporate the positive aspects while discouraging negative aspects of self-help. The group has the benefit of input and support from the workers, but group members may take a larger role in the planning and running of the group.

Assessment

When getting together a group of clients ready to attend a WITHDRAW course the worker needs to have a clear idea of what he is assessing for. The process, whatever the method and content of the assessment, should include certain elements. Before a course starts the worker will have (a) made an initial contact with the client, (b) accepted the client for the group, (c) taken some kind of history or personal details, and (d) planned what kind of course he is going to run.

First contact

The first contact with a client, whether by dropping in, by telephone, or by letter, serves two functions. It provides an opportunity for the worker to gain an impression of the client, to establish the beginnings of rapport, and is often a moment when valuable information can be obtained which may be useful later. It is helpful therefore if initial enquiries whether in person or by telephone can rapidly be channelled to the worker who is going to make the assessment. The client may not yet be committed further than a general enquiry, but the quality of that first contact can influence whether the client decides to proceed further and make an appointment to come and 'have a chat'.

The second function of the first contact is that it gives the client her first impression of the worker and the agency. The receptionist's manner is important, especially in not taking a long list of biographical details and filling in forms which can be off-putting. Appropriate action needs to be taken before the client has got very far with describing the problem or help she requires. This might include passing the client on to the appropriate worker or taking a telephone number and assuring the client she will be called back, giving the worker's name.

The object of the first contact for the worker is to try to get the client to say what help she wants, to describe something of the history, including the drugs she is taking, and, if it seems that the agency can accept this client, to offer an appointment for further discussion.

Some people are quite resistant to making a commitment at this stage, and the worker may need to say the client is under no obligation to proceed further. Some people are under a lot of pressure from doctors, relatives or friends to come off tranquillisers, and need to have their fears or resentment recognised.

Agoraphobia is fairly common as a side-effect of tranquillisers and also as part of the withdrawal syndrome for those who have been reducing on their own, and may be part of the reason why a client may say that she cannot come for an assessment. Persuasion is rarely effective, but recognition of the fears, reassurance that others have coped with their fears and come, and an invitation to bring a friend or discuss travel arrangements may help the client to make this important step.

The assessment interview

The appointment made for an assessment should be confirmed in writing as soon as possible, not only because it can be forgotten, but because it reinforces the decision that the client has made to get some help with coming off tranquillisers. Sending a brief questionnaire at this stage to be returned before the interview continues the process begun in the first contact, of taking the history. The question is what to include and what to leave for the interview itself. Some of the following help to focus the client's thinking about her previous, current, and future tranquilliser use:

(i) Biographical details.
(ii) Current medication.
(iii) Previous drug history.
(iv) Original reasons for taking tranquillisers.
(v) Reasons for continuing to take tranquillisers.
(vi) Reasons for wanting to come off tranquillisers.
(vii) Previous experiences of attempting to come off.

Reading this questionnaire before the interview gives the worker an opportunity to check drug interactions or research difficult questions, and also highlights areas which need to be explored further with the client in the interview.

The worker should begin by making a statement about confidentiality, not only because the client may be concerned about what will happen to what she says and what is written down, but also because it enables the client to speak about quite private matters, if she wishes, before the group meets. Many groups are sabotaged by clients dropping out having made themselves too vulnerable by disclosing private details in a group, or disclosing too soon. This kind of intimate detail can be accepted and contained by the worker, and it is often an important indicator of the level of rapport which is established and the commitment of the client to work with the group leader.

A semi-structured interview works well since it keeps the worker in charge of the interview, monitoring the time, making an assessment of the suitability of the client for various options, while still allowing flexibility in further exploration of issues with the client. The interview may terminate with an offer of treatment, a contract being agreed or some kind of agreement about the next step which both parties will take. It is important for the worker to recognise that this one interview may be the start of the treatment itself, which will continue later in the WITHDRAW group. It may even be the whole intervention if the offer is one of information and advice only, which the client accepts.

The letter which follows the interview to the client should include some feedback to her of the discussion which took place, indicating the worker's view of it, confirmation of any offer of further treatment (for example, a place in a WITHDRAW group), and information about what will happen next. Feedback at this stage increases the take-up rate and enables commitment to be maintained while waiting for the group to start. For those agencies which receive and accept referrals within the National Health Service or from other professional sources, a letter may need to be written to the referrer and the client's general practitioner. A letter to the general practitioner may explain what the client has decided to do, helps to establish co-operation between the doctor and the agency, and seeks the practitioner's support for the client.

What is the worker looking for?

It is important to notice expressions of ambivalence about taking tranquillisers. There may be an assumption that expressions of ambivalence indicate poor motivation but this is not the case. Clients who come with categorical statements about the efficacy of tablets or who want better, non-addictive ones, or other quick-acting therapy, or those who deny that they have, and ever had, any benefit from the drugs, are not likely to have a good outcome.

A second feature to look for is whether the client has any insight into why they are still taking the tranquillisers. Reasons which centre wholly on chemical dependence, poor quality drugs, inherited tendencies and irresponsible prescribing are all indicators that the client is failing or refusing to recognise her part in it. If no responsibility is accepted for taking, then responsibility for coming off is also likely to be shifted on to some other person.

If the treatment option, for which the worker is assessing, is a group programme, then it is important to assess the client's interpersonal skills. Signs that the client finds it difficult to maintain eye contact, is reluctant to speak, and has poor rapport, may indicate that her chances of being able to take part and benefit from group experience are slight. It is reasonable to expect that the client is anxious and tense at the thought of coming to the interview, may be depressed, and may feel quite shy about talking about herself. These factors, as well as the ability to control speech and behaviour, need to be taken into account when assessing for a group.

Who needs more than this?

While assessing clients for a fairly intensive short course in tranquilliser withdrawal, the worker has to bear in mind those who might be acceptable in terms of motivation, insight and sociability but who will need more than such a short course may offer. Different treatment options which may be available include a long-term group, continued support, referral to a more specialist agency, or a more experienced therapist. What should the worker be looking for in these cases?

Some clients may have had help in the past, either from the agency or a self-help group, or other health professionals, and have reduced but not been able to come off their tranquillisers. The indications here are of limited success; that perhaps several stages in the process have been achieved but that new goals can now be explored.

Clients who describe having seen psychiatrists, psychologists, and other professionals in the past, *and have found it useful*, may be involved in a longer process of more fundamental change of which tranquilliser withdrawal is a part. Sometimes the client is aware of needing 'something more' than a short-term withdrawal course. Statements which indicate that the client is aware of some personal issue, such as relationship difficulties or other dependencies, that they need to look at in order to come off tranquillisers are also an indication that more than a short course is appropriate. If a short course is all that is on offer, the worker needs to be realistic in setting goals with the client which are attainable in the time, so that the client does not have unrealistic expectations which will be unfulfilled.

Who might I not accept?

Some agencies will have a policy which excludes certain clients from being accepted for treatment but, where there is some flexibility or a range of options is available, the worker assessing a client needs to be aware of criteria which would tend to exclude clients from short-term withdrawal groups.

Evidence of a wider range of drug use such as anti-psychotic drugs, tranquillisers used with alcohol, tranquillisers used with serious illegal drugs, or a history of alcoholism, compulsive gambling, or other addictive behaviour, indicates possible exclusion. Use of anti-depressants, beta-blockers, or similar symptomatic medication, need not exclude clients from short-term groups. While not particularly helpful, these do not make withdrawal necessarily more difficult, as long as they are not introduced immediately before or during withdrawal, hence disturbing stability.

Some clients will have long-standing involvement with a wide variety of helping agencies and it is important to question the client's ability or willingness to be helped. Statements about the other agencies being no good suggest that the worker is being set up as the next 'expert' to disappoint or let them down.

Socially-isolated clients without an adequate support network to confirm the shift the client is making from user to non-user, or those living in a hostel, may have a poor chance of benefiting from a short-term group. During the assessment it is important to notice whether the client is able to show emotion, or speaks in a detached or stilted way, or seems cut off.

Finally, it is important to consider whether to exclude those who are being pressured, by their spouse, family, or general practitioner, to continue. Statements such as, 'My husband makes me take them', or, 'My doctor says I'm a born worrier', indicate that the client's attempts to withdraw are likely to be sabotaged. On the other hand pressure to withdraw is also likely to be counter-productive. If the client is coming to the assessment because she has been sent by the general practitioner, psychiatrist, or social worker, and is under duress to come off, this pressure needs to be extensively explored, so that the client feels able to make an independent decision.

Keeping the client involved

Writing a letter to the patient and giving her a booklet about waiting for the group to start are important ways of keeping the client involved. The choice of an open group into which a client can immediately be introduced sounds very attractive but there is often much greater benefit to be gained from the changes which the client starts to make, both in thinking and acting, before the group starts. The disadvantages of a wait of several weeks can be minimised by helping the client perceive ways in which she can start to prepare the ground.

The worker also needs time to consider the assessments made in order to write to the general practitioner, or other referrer, to fix dates, times, and a place for the group to meet. Practical problems in getting a group together such as avoiding public holidays which might interrupt the course, and ensuring there is sufficient administrative back up are often under-estimated. Collecting equipment, handouts, booklets, and arranging sessions for supervision, all need to be done before the course starts.

Management of withdrawal

Forming the group

When twelve clients (aim for perhaps eight women and four men) have been assessed as suitable for a short-term group and put on the waiting list, the worker is ready to plan the day, time, and place, where the course will be held. Letters giving all the dates and offering a place should be sent out at least fourteen days in advance to allow time for arrangements to be made for child-minding or time off work. It is important to give the client a leaflet outlining the course which helps to allay fears about whether they have to talk about themselves or come off their tranquillisers during the course, and what will happen when the course ends. Requiring clients to telephone their acceptance of a place tends to reinforce their commitment. A group usually consists of eight to ten people – fewer than this poses some awkward questions about the quality of the assessment!

Aims of the group

Tranquilliser users may already have watched television programmes, read several books, and received quite a lot of help and advice. Rather than a solely intellectual approach, what they may need is an *experience* which addresses their thinking, feeling, and behaviour, in an integrated way. The WITHDRAW group uses a variety of approaches but two main therapeutic bases: cognitive-behaviour therapy and transactional analysis.

The WITHDRAW approach of using an experience to bring about change provides the opportunity to have:

- a feeling of being listened to;
- information and a chance to discuss it;
- a framework to make sense of it;
- a shared experience with others;
- increased confidence and self-esteem;
- skills for living for the future.

The WITHDRAW course

The eight sessions each have a focus and are followed up by homework to practise applying what has been learnt in the session. Most sessions have written material for each group member to take away to remind, reinforce, and practise new learning. This has the advantage of being available for clients to refer to later and to give family and friends an idea of the changes the client is making. Advice, particularly on managing withdrawal, may easily be forgotten, but a ready reference source encourages the client to look for solutions to her difficulties herself.

Session 1 – Introduction

Introductory exercise, information about tranquillisers and how they affect the body, monitoring of clients' use of tranquillisers and other drugs and learning about signs of tension.

Session 2 – Stress and anxiety

Review, information about stress, what goes wrong, alternative ways to deal with stress, relaxation through breathing and deep muscle relaxation.

Session 3 – Withdrawal

Review, guidelines for withdrawal '*at your own pace*', thinking about withdrawal, ways to cope, individual withdrawal programmes.

Session 4 – Positive thinking

Review, introduction to catching, challenging, and changing negative thinking, accepting positive strokes, a positive view of oneself.

Session 5 – Getting to know yourself

Review, introduction to 'parent adult child' (transactional analysis) examining messages from the parent, exercise to develop free child, examining negative strokes.

Session 6 – Getting more out of life

Review, strategies for minimising stress, improving diet and exercise, developing leisure activities and strong personal relationships.

Session 7 – Sabotage

Review, particularly withdrawal and checking negative thinking, introducing sabotaging exercises to promote awareness of sabotage by self and others.

Session 8 – Projections

Review, endings and beginnings, recapitulation of what has been covered, exercise self-help, projections into the future, support in the future, letting go.

Session follow-up

Twelve weeks after the eighth session the group is invited to return, usually on the same day, at the same time, and in the same place. It is important to give the date for this at the end of session eight of the course, and to write at least two weeks in advance to remind group members of the date, enclosing a drug diary for one week for them to complete and bring to the session. It is useful to suggest that clients might like to consider:

(a) what further help they need in coming off or staying off tranquillisers;
(b) what other problem they might need to deal with before coming off completely;
(c) if they are off tranquillisers, what might be their next step.

Aspects of running a group

Before starting a group the worker needs to consider how he will be supported. An important part of working effectively with this type of theme-based group is to recognise that the worker is not going to deal with many of the issues which clients will raise. In fact each group member will be doing at least half of the process outside the group itself. This means that unresolved difficult issues and feelings may be left over at the end of the group for the group leader. For example, clients often feel quite angry about being prescribed tranquillisers in the first place, particularly if they were not warned about side effects, long-term use, or withdrawal. Anger, resentment and frustration may be directed at doctors, nurses, drug companies, and other agencies. The worker cannot resolve these feelings for the client. This needs to be acknowledged and dealt with by the group leader and his co-workers, so that the worker is able to separate himself from the feelings which the session has aroused in him. A 'safe place' for the worker to de-brief and express his feelings is essential if the worker is not to become so overburdened that he is unable to start afresh with each session.

Group leader's guidelines for managing withdrawal

An important feature of the WITHDRAW approach is that the client is the person who is in charge of her withdrawal, and therefore the setting of targets for reducing by either the worker or the general practitioner may not be appropriate. Although superficially it seems helpful to set goals and targets for the client, it has been our experience that this may not be the best method. In general, the control of giving medication has been in the hands of a third party who makes all the decisions over prescribing medication, what type, what dose, when to take it, etc.

The client has played a more passive role in receiving the medication and complying with instructions for use. Whilst the short-term aim is to withdraw from medication, the long-term goal is to remain abstinent. To achieve the latter aim it is important that the client accepts responsibility for her tranquilliser use and hence its reduction. This is achieved partly by regaining some psychological control throughout the withdrawal process. It might take longer, but during a gradual reduction at her own pace, a client is able to learn new coping skills and strategies and gain confidence in her own abilities to reduce dependence on tranquillisers. This is crucial for continued abstinence. The worker is there to provide information, support, and to negotiate a reasonable reduction rather than to break down the client's resistance or encourage any passivity.

Some people are too anxious to make progress and may set themselves unreasonable targets, sabotaging themselves or feeling guilty if the expected reduction rate is not achieved. Equally, if targets are set by another person it can provoke resistance, 'game playing' around meeting targets, or simply reinforce the person's dependence on external sources to solve problems. In our experience anti-depressants and beta-blockers do not generally aid withdrawal, and may reinforce dependence on medication as a coping strategy.

1. Stabilise on the same dose at the same time each day for about two weeks. Take by the clock – not by how you feel.
2. Decide which is the least needed tablet.
3. Choose a good time – not in the middle of a crisis.
4. Reduce only one tranquilliser at a time.
5. Leave anti-depressants and beta-blockers until later.
6. Reduce one dose by not more than one eighth of total daily dose.
7. Wait at least two weeks until any withdrawal effect will have happened.
8. If the withdrawal syndrome occurs – stick it out! Find other ways to cope.
9. Wait until comfortable and confident again before making another reduction.
10. Remember withdrawal effects will pass in time.

Further details on managing withdrawal can be found in the leaflet 'Gently does it' (WITHDRAW Project 1987).

Some research findings

Half-lives and breakdown products

Tranquillisers are frequently categorised by their length of action, the half-life being the length of time it takes for the amount of drug in the blood to be halved. Several things can affect the amount of a drug in the blood – the time of day when the drug is taken, body weight, whether taken before or after a meal, age, and the daily dose. Some of the breakdown products which are produced are also clinically active and continue to have a tranquillising effect.

People taking tranquillisers with a long half-life are unlikely to experience withdrawal effects between doses but may feel continually tired or drowsy. Those taking a tranquilliser with a short or medium half-life are likely to experience withdrawal between doses. This is frequently the case with short-acting hypnotics, the withdrawal effects of which can wake people up in the middle of the night – a self-defeating drug! People taking short- or medium-acting tranquillisers in one daily dose may feel the withdrawal effects first thing in the morning and not be aware that they are withdrawing.

It is possible to categorise tranquillisers by the duration of action (Trickett 1986): the duration of action affects the length of time before withdrawal symptoms occur, and also the length of time the withdrawal is experienced (see Table 7.1).

Table 7.1 Duration of action of various tranquillisers

Long-acting	*Medium*	*Short*
diazepam	temazepam	oxazepam
chlordiazepoxide	lorazepam	triazolam (very short)
nitrazepam		

Source: Trickett 1986.

The withdrawal syndrome

The syndrome may begin within the first two to three days or be delayed for seven to fourteen days; it increases in severity and reaches a peak before diminishing until it is finally resolved and the symptoms have gone away. Evidence about the duration of the syndrome shows that this can take from two to three weeks (Owen and Tyrer 1983) to two to three months (Schopf 1983).

It may be quite difficult to distinguish between anxiety symptoms, side effects, and the withdrawal syndrome. We have found that people experiencing withdrawal symptoms start their tranquillisers again because they believe that the original anxiety is resurfacing. There is evidence that some symptoms such as sore gums and increased sensitivity to light or sound are uncharacteristic of anxiety (Petursson and Lader 1981; Owen and Tyrer 1983). The withdrawal syndrome is also described by MacKinnon and Parker (1982) who divide symptoms into mild and severe. Symptoms are classed as mild if they are mainly perceptual changes, and as severe if they are mainly physiological changes.

A summary of the symptoms of withdrawal listed in five categories is given by Schopf (1983). The main experiences seem to be:

irritability
lack of energy
poor memory
difficulty concentrating
influenza-like illness
seeing things
depression
unusual effects from alcohol and caffeine
muscle pain
nausea
digestive difficulties
shakiness
perspiration
poor co-ordination
sleeping difficulties
metallic taste

It is important to recognise that some or any of these symptoms can be very severe, particularly if the withdrawal is too rapid and the person has not stabilised following one reduction when another reduction is made. Since individuals vary from each other, and the syndrome may vary for a particular person each time a reduction is made, the only safe way to ensure the withdrawal syndrome is manageable is to make small reductions and to wait for the syndrome to subside before the next reduction is made. It is usually inadvisable for anyone to stop taking tranquillisers suddenly even if 'getting it over quickly' seems an attractive idea. Abrupt withdrawal increases the risk of very severe symptoms which include convulsions, hallucinations, and psychotic episodes.

We have had clients who have previously withdrawn too abruptly and sought help in desperation for acute depression or other severe symptoms. The syndrome may be difficult to recognise if the client does not connect her symptoms with abrupt tranquilliser withdrawal. Alternative medication for symptomatic relief may confirm the client's and her family's fears that she is going mad or is about to die.

Understandably, such previous experiences make further attempts to withdraw difficult, and the reassurance that withdrawal can be made manageable, and at the client's own pace, is crucial. Not only is the relationship with the worker important in these cases, but also the fact that withdrawal is understood and alternative ways of coping have been learned *before* withdrawal is attempted.

How soon does the syndrome start?

How soon the withdrawal syndrome starts is partly dependent upon the half-life of the tranquilliser being taken, and whether other benzodiazepines are also being used (for example, hypnotics). If the half-life is shorter (that is, less than twelve hours), then a person may experience withdrawal between doses. However, if the tranquilliser is longer acting, then withdrawal can start within three to ten days of any reduction (Committee on the Review of Medicines 1980). In practice, there is such a wide individual variation that at least fourteen days should be allowed before consideration is given to any further reduction. If the withdrawal syndrome does occur, then no further reduction should be made until the symptoms of withdrawal have passed. An exception to this occurs when taking shorter-acting tranquillisers in very low dose, when almost constant withdrawal is experienced. The final reduction to coming off completely can usually be considered after about three weeks from the previous reduction.

Should people transfer to longer-acting tranquillisers?

The longer a person has been taking tranquillisers before reducing, the higher the chances that tolerance and dependence have developed. Tyrer *et al.* (1981) suggest that the rate of decrease of tranquillisers in the blood determines whether withdrawal symptoms are experienced. They suggest changing to a longer-acting tranquilliser to ensure a more gradual decrease. If this is done it is recommended that the transfer is done one dose at a time every two to three days, and that care is taken to maintain equivalent doses (Ashton 1984).

In practice, this is more difficult than it sounds. There are no exact equivalents, and some symptoms of withdrawal may be experienced even when transferring from one tranquilliser to another, and larger doses may be needed. Switches to longer-acting tranquillisers, or anti-depressants, or beta-blockers, as aids to withdrawal because they are 'easier to withdraw from' may not necessarily be helpful. Attempts to find easier pharmacological methods of withdrawal are important but psychological dependence on tranquillisers should not be overlooked. Switching to other drugs may be in conflict with giving an underlying message to the client that she can learn alternative methods of coping without recourse to medication.

Effect of the length of time on tranquillisers

Taking short- or medium-acting hypnotics for one or two nights can result in 'rebound insomnia' when the drug is withdrawn (Kales *et al.* 1979). Longer-acting tranquillisers in normal dose can induce dependence in two to three months (Covi *et al.* 1973). An indication of the proportion of people who could be expected to develop withdrawal symptoms according to the length of time taken is given by Petursson and Lader (1984) (see Table 7.2).

However, people taking higher doses (two to five times therapeutic doses) are likely to develop dependence within two to three weeks of use (Petursson 1982). Petursson also found that, although the rate of first-time users of tranquillisers is falling, the average length of time people are taking them is increasing. This is worrying since the length of duration of drug use may be one of the most important factors in determining the risk of dependence.

One way of estimating the likelihood and severity of the withdrawal syndrome (which should affect time taken to withdraw) is to use the Cumulative Benzodiazepine Exposure Index developed by Busto *et al.* (1986) which measures a person's total tranquilliser

Table 7.2 The prevalence of withdrawal symptoms with different durations of use

Length of use (therapeutic dosage)	*% people experiencing withdrawal*
Less than 4 months	Rarely – except short-acting tranx
6–12 months	5–10
1–2 years	No figures (? 15–20)
2–4 years	25–45
6–8 years	75

Source: Petursson and Lader 1984.

intake. It is calculated by multiplying dosage by index value and by duration of use.

An index of sedative strength gives approximate equivalent doses to diazepam (see Table 7.3).

Table 7.3 The relative sedative strength of various tranquillisers

Tranquilliser		*Index*	*Equivalent in diazepam*
diazepam	10mg	1	10mg
chlordiazepoxide	30mg	0.5	15mg
lorazepam	3mg	10	30mg
oxazepam	30mg	0.3	10mg
nitrazepam	5mg	1	5mg
temazepam	20mg	0.5	10mg
triazolam	0.125mg	20	2.5mg

Source: WITHDRAW Project 1987.

Conclusion

Any worker involved in managing tranquilliser withdrawal needs to keep abreast of developments taking place elsewhere. There is a national Benzodiazepine Interest Group which produces a newsletter providing a useful way for workers to exchange ideas and information about tranquilliser withdrawal. Past experience teaches us the importance of attending to the first warning signs of problems with new drugs. Benzodiazepines are unlikely to be the only prescribed medication which have associated difficulties, nor are the problems which this group of drugs presents fully understood yet.

If tranquillisers are no longer seen as a long-term solution to anxiety and stress-related problems, then what is? Much of the experience gained in managing withdrawal points to fruitful areas of investigation in the search for alternatives. Alternative medication will act as a stopgap until non-medical approaches are developed. No doubt a whole range of possible interventions needs to be explored, tried, tested, and evaluated, to meet the varied needs of clients.

References

Ashton, H. (1984) 'Benzodiazepine withdrawal: an unfinished story', *British Medical Journal*, 288: 1135–40.

Busto, U., Sellers, E.M., Naranjo, C.A., Cappell, H.D., Sanchez-Craig, M., and Simpkins, J. (1986) 'Patterns of benzodiazepine abuse and dependence', *British Journal of Addiction*, 81: 87–94.

Committee on the Review of Medicines (1980) 'Systematic review of the benzodiazepines', *British Medical Journal*, 280: 910–12.

Committee on the Safety of Medicines (1988) ' Benzodiazepines, dependence and withdrawal symptoms', *Current Problems*, no. 21 (January).

Covi, L., Lipman, R.S., Pattison, J.H., Derogatis, L.R., and Uhlenhuth, E.H. (1973) 'Length of treatment with anxiolytic sedatives and response to their sudden withdrawal', *Acta psychiatrica scandanavica*, 49: 51–64.

Hamlin, M. (1988) 'An integrated cognitive behavioural approach to withdrawal from tranquillisers', in Dryden, W. and Trower, P. (eds) *Developments in Cognitive Psychotherapy*, London: Sage Publications.

Kales, A., Scharf, M.B., Kales, J.D., Constantin, R., and Soldatos, R. (1979) 'Rebound insomnia. A potential hazard following withdrawal of certain benzodiazepines', *Journal of the Americam Medical Association*, 241 (16): 1692–5.

MacKinnon, G.L. and Parker, W.A. (1982) 'Benzodiazepine withdrawal syndrome: a literature review and evaluation', *American Journal of Drug and Alcohol Abuse*, 9 (1): 19–33.

Owen, R.T. and Tyrer, P. (1983) 'Benzodiazepine dependence: a review of the evidence', *Drugs*, 25: 385–98.

Petursson, H. (1982) 'Clinical and laboratory studies of withdrawal from long-term benzodiazepine treatment', PhD thesis, London: Institute of Psychiatry.

Petursson, H. and Lader, M.H. (1981) 'Withdrawal from long-term benzodiazepines treatment', *British Medical Journal*, 283: 643–5.

Petursson, H. and Lader, M.H. (1984) *Dependence on Tranquillisers*, Institute of Psychiatry: Maudsley Monographs, no. 28, Oxford University Press.

Royal College of Psychiatrists (1988) 'Benzodiazepines and dependence: a college statement', *Bulletin of the Royal College of Psychiatrists*, 12: 107–13.

Schopf, J. (1983) 'Withdrawal phenomena after long-term administration of benzodiazepines. A review of recent investigations', *Pharmacopsychiatry*, 16: 1–8.

Trickett, S. (1986) *Coming off Tranquillisers: A Withdrawal Plan that really works*, Wellingborough: Thorsons.

Tyrer, P., Rutherford, D., and Higgett, T. (1981) 'Benzodiazepine withdrawal symptoms and propanolol', *The Lancet*, 1: 520–2.

WITHDRAW Project (1986) *Aspects of Withdrawal from Benzodiazepines – A guide for those who work with tranquilliser withdrawal*, WITHDRAW Project, North Birmingham Health Authority.

WITHDRAW Project (1987) 'Gently does it', WITHDRAW Project, North Birmingham Health Authority.

Chapter Eight

Facing up to AIDS

Stewart Dickson and Jane Hollis

This chapter discusses the problem of Human Immunosuppressive Virus/Acquired Immune Deficiency Syndrome (HIV/AIDS) in relation to drug abusers and how the risks of infection in this group can be reduced. It deals with how to counsel people before and after an antibody test, and looks at the working environment and the future prospects for drug agencies.

Introduction

Drug abusers have never bothered about hepatitis, overdoses, choking to death on their own vomit, thrombosis, gangrene or heroin cut with strychnine – so why should they worry about AIDS? The fact that more and more drug abusers are being identified as HIV-positive is unlikely to influence them.

AIDS is potentially the most serious sociomedical situation facing us at present. In the words of the World Health Organisation: 'We are for the first time in history at the beginning of a plague'.

At the beginning of the AIDS scare, the main risk groups were identified as homosexual men, drug abusers, and recipients of infected blood. The homosexual community have responded to information campaigns quickly and responsibly. Research by doctors from the Middlesex University College Hospital points to a change to safer sexual practices which is already leading to a slowdown in the rise of HIV infection (Anon 1987a). A study of homosexual and bisexual men attending the Middlesex Hospital sexually transmitted diseases (STD) clinic found that between 1982 and 1984 the number who were seropositive rose by 7.4 per cent a year. But by December 1986 this increase had fallen to 1.8 per cent. The slower rise in antibody positive men coincided with a fall in the annual rate of gonorrhoea from 15.3 per cent in 1982 to only 5.1 per cent in the first half of 1986.

All donated blood in the western world is now tested and heat-treated to destroy the HIV virus and is safe. The spread of the virus through heterosexual intercourse has been massively publicised through a government funded media campaign and noone is now likely to 'die of ignorance'. But many drug abusers don't care about dying, and they continue to spread infection by sharing needles and – even more dangerously – through sex. Many drug abusers, both male and female, resort to prostitution to fund their habits, and thus pass the infection on into the wider community.

The problem

Risks of drug users

Drug abusers have a very poor record of looking after themselves physically or of being aware of health, diet, and general and sexual hygiene. They generally tend to have a rather negative, sometimes nihilistic view of themselves, their lives, and relationships. This is an attitudinal problem which all of us working with drug abusers have had to confront and work with in our relationships with clients, as we have tried to steer them towards a healthier life-style.

The battle with many drug abusers to get them to stop abusing drugs, or to take a methadone script, is very difficult. With the spread of HIV among drug abusers, we are now having to embark on major education programmes, particularly in the areas of safer sex and general hygiene. Our client groups are going to need a great deal of basic information on HIV/AIDS, on how to prepare needles and syringes hygienically, the availability of needle exchange schemes, and the dangers of needle sharing. Couple this with a sex education programme and we are facing a very difficult task.

Needle sharing

There is little research so far published on the significance of HIV/AIDS on needle-sharing practices. However, it does seem that differences in the prevalence of sharing needles affects the incidence of HIV. This is especially obvious in Scotland, where the spread of infection has been rapid. Sixty-four per cent of reported HIV infected people are drug abusers. A report from the Scottish Committee on HIV infection and Intravenous Drug Misuse (Scottish Home and Health Department 1986) blames in part 'the emphasis of police activity . . . on discouraging the sale of syringes and needles, and removing these items from individuals found in possession of them'. This emphasis has led to a tradition of 'shooting galleries' in Scotland where addicts can use a communal syringe and needle to inject their drugs.

Anecdotal evidence suggests that there is becoming a higher awareness of the danger of sharing needles. Some of the clients in our own unit say they stopped sharing needles some time ago. These reports are confirmed by more extensive surveys.

Ghodse *et al.* (1987) looked at the injection practices of 232 drug users attending three London drug-dependency treatment units in January 1987. Of 150 respondents who thought they had received sufficient information about AIDS, 83 per cent had consequently changed their drug-using habits, either by not injecting or not sharing. Strang *et al.* (1987), in a follow-up study after two to three years, found that, out of 55 continuing drug users, 42 per cent had reduced the frequency of injecting (20 per cent had stopped injecting). A recent study carried out in Edinburgh found that intravenous drug users reported substantial decreases in needle sharing over the course of a year (Robertson *et al.* 1988). Together these studies show that injecting drug users can reduce these high-risk behaviours. These results should encourage agencies to work with those who do not wish to stop using drugs, with the goal of harm reduction.

We have always viewed drug abuse as being a social/cultural activity. This makes it very difficult to break some of the needle-sharing rituals and habits that are already formed and established in intravenous (IV) drug abuse groups. It is important to remember that you cannot realistically ask anyone to change a behavioural pattern unless you can offer them an alternative that is acceptable to them.

There are two major alternatives to sharing needles – abstinence, and the supply of free needles. Not all drug abusers can achieve total abstinence, and many do not even want to. The supply of free needles is essential to ensure that anyone who has not yet reached the stage of being able to give up drugs can at least minimise the risks.

Reducing risks

Safer drug use

Most people who work with drug abusers are aiming in the long term to help their clients stop taking drugs. However, this may take years and there is much we can do in the meantime to minimise the risk that they may not live long enough to reach the point where they are ready to do this. Counselling in the area of HIV and AIDS is simply another aspect of this work.

Intravenous drug abusers may make up a small part of our overall drug abuse clientele, therefore it is easy to identify this group, single them out for special attention, and miss the fact that clients using methods other than intravenous injection are also in an exceedingly vulnerable situation; they are at risk of being infected by HIV when their judgement is impaired by drugs. Although IV drug abusers need special counselling, it is very important that we do not forget the risk to all our clients, including those dependent on legal drugs such as tranquillisers and alcohol.

Injecting drug abusers

Some injecting users may be willing, after counselling, to change to an oral method. If not, they need information about how they can inject safely. Access to sterile injecting equipment is necessary for safe injections. Where access is limited, some drug takers will attempt to sterilise their 'works'.

Sterilising injection equipment

The Terence Higgins Trust has published a leaflet telling drug users how to sterilise their 'works'. This is the only way it is safe to share 'works' (Table 8.1).

This is an ideal procedure. Yet, we have to remember that many of our clients will not be in a physical condition to go through this procedure, they will fumble it, will in some cases miss out sections of it, or not bother with it at all. It is a very lengthy and complicated procedure for someone who is waiting on a hit.

The latest advice from the Standing Conference on Drug Abuse is that the use of bleach is not recommended, as it tends to harden dried blood and therefore may protect the virus. Bleach may also corrode the metal parts of the syringe, making it harder to clean away traces of blood. The current recommendation is that 'works' should be flushed out as soon as possible after use with several changes of clean cold water to which a small amount of washing-up liquid has been added. This advice, too, may be superseded in the future.

The only really safe way of injecting drugs is to use a completely new set of 'works' every time. If this is not possible, advise clients to keep their 'works' safe and not mix them up with those belonging to other people. When they have finished with the 'works' they should destroy them in a way that no one else can use them or be accidentally pricked by the needle. This is especially important if there are children around. They should not mix their fix in a spoon that someone else has used, or flush out their 'works' with water which someone else has already used to clean theirs.

It is important to stress to clients that it is never safe to share syringes or needles, even with close friends. You can never be sure who may have the virus, or be exposing themselves to infection elsewhere (through injection or sexually).

Table 8.1 How to clean your 'works'

1. Take the syringe to pieces.
2. Under running water, scrub it inside and out with a toothbrush (if possible other than the one used for brushing teeth).
3. Get some household bleach, like DOMESTOS – Dettol, Savlon or other disinfectants do not work against this virus.
4. Get a large bowl.
5. Use 1 part of bleach to 9 parts of water.
6. Take the syringe to pieces. Put all the bits into the bleach solution, and leave them for as long as you can, preferably at least half an hour.

Now rinse all the pieces together in warm running water at least five times, you must get rid of all the bleach solution from the 'works' before you use them. Do not repeat this more than a couple of times as bleach will eventually corrode the metal needle. Get a new set.

Needle-exchange schemes

The DHSS have currently set up twelve pilot needle-exchange schemes in this country with a view to monitoring their use and effectiveness. There are a number of pros and cons and arguments concerning needle-exchange schemes. Our primary concern is the criteria for issuing the needles. Should needles just be issued to anyone on demand? This may facilitate the spread of injecting, moving groups of people from smoking heroin, snorting amphetamines or cocaine into injecting because of the easy availability of needles. In conjunction with this, most people injecting would be more relaxed in their habits and HIV may further spread through those areas.

The opposing viewpoint to this is that if needles are available freely to any individual who wants them, there will be such a flood of clean needles that the spread through needle sharing will be reduced.

There has been a generally favourable report on some of the needle-exchange schemes which have been set up. One of the early envisaged problems was the relationship between the police and the needle schemes, but in some areas this seems to have been overcome in a sympathetic and logical way. For example, a letter in *The Lancet* (Marks and Parry 1987) reports that the Merseyside Police Drugs Squad have co-operated with the area needle-exchange policy in two ways. When an addict is arrested but not detained, s/he is given a leaflet about the risk of AIDS and about the needle-sharing scheme. The police also operate a policy of not waiting outside the exchange to arrest addicts. This is an effort to encourage addicts to seek help without fear of retribution.

The Mersey Regional Drugs Training and Information Centre, which has been offering free needles and syringes to IV users since October 1986, is optimistic about the success of its scheme – general health, return of used equipment, and level of information among clients have all improved. In addition, 50 per cent of clients had no previous contact with any treatment agency, and thus more people at risk are being reached (Carr 1987).

Reports from Amsterdam indicate that providing clean needles has not encouraged injecting. In 1985, 100,000 syringes were provided on an exchange basis and the number of addicts injecting did not increase (25 to 30 per cent inject, 70 to 75 per cent inhale or smoke). Therapeutic programmes report that more clients than ever are entering treatment (Buning *et al.* 1986).

In America, education programmes on needle sharing and risk reduction in general for drug users do not so far appear effective. A British worker in the field who visited the USA in 1986 on a fellowship concludes:

> My experience in the USA left me feeling sad and frustrated. The USA could learn from the UK experience of embracing the AIDS issue. In September the public health campaign in the USA had yet to begin. Major risks were being taken in the USA by not making the public aware. No-one seems to be prepared to take the positive risk of providing a hard hitting, straight talking campaign in case offence is caused to some sector of American society. It was being said that American hospitals were making contingency plans to turn away AIDS sufferers in the event of saturation. In comparison, it is important that we give credit to the much more positive action taken by the Department of Health and Social Security.
>
> (Martin 1986)

More information is needed about the efficacy of needle-exchange schemes – and for this to happen, more schemes need to be set up. If they prove a failure, we may see extreme legal sanctions on IV drug abusers possessing illegal equipment.

Guidelines for a needle-exchange scheme set up in the Portsmouth area in 1987, plus notes for users, are given in Tables 8.2 and 8.3.

Finally, we would like to reiterate our own view, that however much we may deplore the abuse of drugs, our primary aim should be to promote a healthier life-style in our clients and minimise the risk of HIV infection.

Table 8.2 Proposals for needles- and syringe-exchange scheme

1. The clinic to be situated at ....
2. The clinic to be open on Monday, Tuesday, Thursday and Friday afternoons for needle/syringe exchange, counselling for HIV and all health aspects.
3. Injecting equipment to be issued on an exchange basis to drug misusers who are already injecting and are unable or unwilling to stop. The service will be open to all injecting drug misusers. Injection sites will be regularly inspected by staff.
4. The number of needles/syringes issued initially to each client to be negotiated at the first interview. Maximum of 10 per visit.
5. Questionnaires to be completed by each client during the first few weeks of contact. The questions will include client's attitudes, knowledge, and behaviour, with regard to drug use and drug-using practices, sexual activity and HIV/AIDS. A further questionnaire would be completed at a period of between two and three months. The questionnaire would take approximately thirty minutes to complete.
6. Information collected to be forwarded to the research team for analysis. To ensure anonymity a unique identifier number to be allocated to each client.
7. Returned needles/syringes to be counted and recorded by staff. A 100 per cent return rate should be aimed for, but it is recognised that this may not always be achievable.
8. Returned needles/syringes to be carried to the clinic by the client in a suitable hard container, for example, tin or plastic box. These will be issued by the clinic if necessary.
9. Returned needles/syringes to be placed in a suitable sharps container which will be removed and replaced according to Area Health Authority regulations.
10. Clients on the exchange scheme would be encouraged to attend regularly and to be provided with counselling and assessment of his/her drug misuse problem and should s/he wish to seek further treatment, to be referred to the Drug Advice Centre at Northern Road Clinic.
11. Counselling to be aimed at ultimately helping the client to stop or reduce his/her drug misuse.
12. Where it is immediately impossible to stop injecting, information about the risks of shared injecting and about safe injecting practices would be provided. It will be clearly stated that the equipment issued is for the client's own use only.
13. Clients would be counselled about the risks of receiving or passing on the AIDS virus by:

    (a) shared injecting practices;
    (b) sexual activity.

    Advice on safer sex to be given and condoms will be available for issue to clients.
14. HIV counselling will be available and testing offered where required.
15. Clients with infected sores or abscesses will be treated in the clinic by nursing staff and will be given advice on sterile techniques of cleansing and dressing wounds. Advice on good general health and diet will be given where required.
16. Clients will have access to a Motivational Group session where there will be coffee facilities available at a minimum cost.
17. Each client will also be seen on an individual basis, in an adjoining room to where the needle/syringe exchange will take place. There will also be the opportunity for individual counselling at this point.
18. Further appointments for counselling will be offered on alternative afternoons if required.

19. Clients already on the Northern Road Clinic Methadone Therapy Programme will not be excluded from the scheme.
20. All clients in the needle/syringe exchange scheme will have the following information recorded: details of contacts, syringes issued and returned, any treatment given and illness episodes.

Table 8.3 Notes for users of needle- and syringe-exchange scheme

1. Please remember that equipment issued is for the sole use of the person it is issued to. DO NOT SHARE.
2. A container has been provided for you to transport your needles and syringes to and from the clinic. Please use it each time.
3. Needles and syringes will only be issued on an exchange basis: one for one. Please keep track of your equipment.
4. Needle and syringe exchange will be available to you on Monday, Tuesday, Thursday and Friday afternoons from 2.30 to 4pm at ....
5. Before disposal, please place all used works in the self-sealing bag provided.
6. If possible, please flush through your equipment with a solution of bleach or Milton.

Safer sex

As well as getting to know the drug history and injecting habits of our clients, we need to talk to them about their sexual activities, and educate them about the need for safer sex.

It is important not to make any assumptions. It is true that many opiate abusers lose their sex drive, but this does not mean they never have sex. They may be regularly financing their habit through prostitution (both male and female). They may occasionally use sex as a means of getting drugs, money, protection, or a place to sleep. Clients in a stable relationship may still occasionally have sexual contact with others, as may their partner. Even in a totally monogamous relationship there is a risk of contracting HIV sexually from a partner who picked it up by sharing needles with an infected person. So anybody who is not absolutely confident that their partners are not infected should be practising safer sex. This 'risk group' includes high numbers of heterosexual non-drug abusers, as well as the clients we are concerned with. In fact, we should not talk about high-risk groups but about high-risk behaviour – sharing needles and not practising safer sex.

We have talked about 'safer sex' – but what exactly does this mean? Basically, any sexual contact that involves the exchange of body fluids is unsafe (the semen, vaginal secretion, blood, and urine of infected people all contain the virus). Unsafe practices become even more unsafe when used repeatedly or together, and the risk increases with the number of different partners:

Vaginal intercourse

Infected semen can enter a woman's bloodstream through her vagina. Pre-ejaculatory fluid may also contain the virus. Infected vaginal secretions can infect a man, especially if there are abrasions (which can be microscopically small) on the penis. Vaginal intercourse can be made safer if a condom is worn throughout contact in such a way as to prevent any exchange of body fluid. The use of a spermicide containing nonoxynol-9 is a further safeguard as this ingredient is thought to destroy the virus.

Anal intercourse

This is even riskier than vaginal intercourse because the lining of the rectum is thin and easily torn. Use of a condom and spermicide as above makes it safer, but condoms are more easily damaged or pulled off than in vaginal intercourse.

Oral sex

This is less risky, but infected semen or vaginal secretions could enter the bloodstream through cuts or sores in the mouth. Oral sex to a man is safer if he wears a condom. Oral sex to a woman is highly unsafe if she is menstruating.

Sado-masochistic practices

Any practice which draws blood is unsafe. Biting, whipping, beating, etc., are safe so long as there is no blood.

Water sports

Sexual practices involving urine (or faeces) are potentially dangerous if body fluids enter another person's body through the eyes, mouth, anus, penis, or vagina, or through cuts anywhere on the body.

Sex toys

It is safe to use sex toys (for example, dildoes, vibrators, dolls) so long as each person has one for his or her own exclusive use. Sharing may pass the infection.

Lesbian sexual practices

There is now evidence (Anon 1987b) of female-to-female transmission of HIV. It is therefore important to remember that women in a lesbian relationship should practise safer sex, avoiding sharing sex toys and sexual practices that cause bleeding of the vulva or vagina.

It is easy to say to clients 'use a condom'. We have to remember that most young people today have never had to use condoms because of the easy availability of the birth control pill and the intrauterine device. We have to educate an entire generation in the proper use of condoms, how to put them on, take them off, and dispose of them safely. This means having condoms in our offices to give to clients and to demonstrate – bananas are a useful resource here! This can also be a good way of lightening the atmosphere a little – sex should be fun. The instructions to give are set out in Table. 8.4.

Table 8.4 How to use condoms

1. Open the packet carefully, ensuring you don't damage the condom with your fingernails.
2. Take hold of the teat end with two fingers to expel the air.
3. Roll the condom down over the erect penis, making sure you roll it right down to the end. If you use a lubricant, apply it after you have the condom on. Use a water-soluble lubricant (KY Jelly or Duragel – vaseline and other oil-based lubricants dissolve the rubber). The condom should be put on before there is any contact between your penis and your partner's body.
4. When inserting the penis, make sure the condom is still in place by feeling for the rim at the base of the penis.
5. After ejaculating, and before the penis becomes limp, withdraw carefully, holding the condom in place. Ensure no semen spills on your partner's body.
6. Remove condom away from your partner's body, wrap it in a tissue. Flush it down the lavatory.
7. Wash the penis before any further contact.
8. Use a new condom each time.
9. Practice makes perfect – and it is a good idea to practise using a condom while masturbating. Using a condom can be more fun when your partner puts it on for you, and by experimenting with all the exotic types now on the market. But make sure you only use condoms that carry the British Standards Institute kitemark.

As mentioned earlier when talking about sharing needles, it is extremely difficult to get someone to change a behavioural pattern without offering an alternative. As counsellors, we need to help our clients discover ways of making love that are exciting, satisfying, fulfilling, and safe.

Having gone through the basic facts about what sexual practices the client uses, and talking about what is not safe, give him or her two large sheets of paper and some felt pens (this is even more effective in a group). Now ask them to write on one sheet all the unsafe practices, and on the other use their imagination and come up with as many safe and exciting sex practices as they can think of. Do two sheets yourself and then compare. Examples – group and mutual masturbation, massage, taking showers and baths together, sexy talk, erotic books and videos, dressing up, sharing and acting-out fantasies, mirrors, polaroid cameras, body rubbing, contact and movement, sex toys (not shared), body kissing and licking away from the genitals, and so on.

Always remind your client that being stoned or drunk may put them at risk sexually.

Women clients need special counselling in view of two facts:

1. Babies born to women who are seropositive (AB+) are often infected too, through the placental exchange of blood. Such babies are highly likely to move into the full AIDS syndrome in the first year because the immune system in the newborn is not fully developed.
2. Pregnancy in itself has been found to be a trigger from HIV infection to AIDS.

Therefore women should not only insist that their partner uses a condom during sexual intercourse, but they should also use some other form of birth control to ensure they do not become pregnant. This is often a problem with drug users because certain drugs (especially barbiturates) can affect the action of the birth control pill, so the cap or coil are safer.

Many women who use drugs cease to menstruate. This does not mean that they are infertile: they should use birth control, even if they do not have periods.

Safer sex counselling is not issuing a list of 'don'ts'. It's talking about sex – and we may first have to examine our own inhibitions, attitudes, and fears. We have to learn to be comfortable and non-judgemental with other people's sexuality which might be different from our own.

The most difficult issue for many people is the use of colloquial language to describe sex organs and sex acts.

Some clients won't understand words like anal intercourse, vagina, semen, cunnilingus, and will feel alienated and resentful if the counsellor talks like that. Anyone who doesn't feel able to use street language like fuck, cock, cum, suck, etc., will need support from colleagues – and that shouldn't be judged either.

Finally, it is essential to note that all these precautions in needle sharing and sexual practices should be taught to your client group in order to guard against the spread of hepatitis and other sexually transmitted diseases. These are not new precautions, and are not solely relevant to HIV and AIDS. They are precautions which have always been largely ignored and are now only highlighted through increased awareness and spread of HIV.

Counselling regarding HIV testing

In October 1985 the DHSS issued guidelines to all doctors in England stating that arrangements should be made to provide pre-test counselling to all patients requesting the test, and post-test counselling for all individuals found to be seropositive (AB+) (DHSS 1985).

Pre-test counselling

The aim of pre-test counselling is two-fold:

1. To ensure that anyone found to be AB+ already has the facts about HIV and AIDS, risk-reduction, health care, etc. This information will have to be repeated after the test result is known, but it is more likely to be properly understood if first presented before the individual is in the state of shock likely to be engendered by a positive result.
2. To make the individual fully aware of the implications of taking the test, and to obtain fully informed consent.

At the first meeting the counsellor should:

1. Ask clients why they wish to be tested. Do they belong to a high-risk group or could they belong to the ever-increasing number of 'worried well'? If the latter, they may need specific counselling.
2. Ascertain what the client thinks the test means and correct any misconceptions. The test is NOT a test for AIDS and there is no such test.
3. Inform clients that advice given about general health care, sexual activity, and the spread of the virus will be the same if the result is positive or negative, or indeed if the test is not performed. Tell the client what this advice is (see post-test counselling below) and provide written material.
4. Inform the client of the arguments for and against having the test:
   (a) Dentists should be told of a positive result, so they can take what precautions they think necessary – but many dentists will then refuse treatment.
   (b) GPs should be told of a positive result so they can watch for signs of ill-health that could be connected to HIV infection. Some GPs respond well, but others ask the Family Practitioner Committee to remove such patients from their list. GPs are often asked to give medical information about

a patient by employers, insurance companies, etc. Not everyone realises that by signing an application form that asks for your GP's name, you are giving consent to the GP to divulge this information.

(c) Employers – many employers discriminate against seropositives and no test case for wrongful dismissal has been brought.

(d) Insurance companies are refusing to insure anyone who is AB+. If a policy is refused, the name of the client may be entered on the 'bad risk' register which is available to banks, credit card companies, etc.

(e) An obvious reason to have the test is to protect sexual partners. But anyone putting themselves at risk should be following safer sex guidelines, and as the virus spreads outside these groups, so should anyone not in a long-term mutually monogamous relationship.

(f) Many people feel that the only way they will be able to follow safer sex and other guidelines is if they know they are AB+. Be aware that these people may treat a negative result as a licence to go on putting themselves and others at risk.

(g) A positive test result usually leads to extreme anxiety and depression. Would the client be able to cope with this? Some people, however, suffer more anxiety from not knowing their antibody status.

(h) An important advantage of taking the test is that people who know they are AB+ can minimise their chances of developing AIDS by strengthening their immune systems with diet, regular exercise and sleep, stress limitation and by reducing smoking, alcohol and drug use.

5. Provide the client with written material to take away, and offer another appointment to discuss his/her decision. Impress upon the client that you will respect whatever decision is made, or be available for further discussion if needed. If the client feels that their decision is contrary to your wishes – that is, if you have failed to remain objective – then they may not come again and you will have lost the opportunity for post-test counselling.

Counselling after a positive result

Be prepared to spend at least an hour on the first session and to offer at least two follow-up sessions. Ensure that you will be able to offer your individual attention and privacy.

The first task is to tell your client clearly and directly that the test result is positive. Later in the session you will have to get several important facts across, but bear in mind that anyone – even if prepared for it – is going to be deeply shocked at the news that s/he is at risk of developing a terminal and incurable illness. Reactions to shock vary, and may include grief, anger, denial, and avoidance. It is essential to allow clients to ventilate these emotions, otherwise they will not be able to free their thinking to listen to information. If no reaction is apparent, then you need to ask, 'How do you feel?' For many people the fear of social isolation and rejection is uppermost, and it can be very reassuring and comforting to be touched as a concrete demonstration of your acceptance.

There is no point in trying to gloss over the fact that AB+ status may lead to AIDS. You can say, however, that not all AB+s develop AIDS, and that there are positive steps to be taken to reduce the risk.

When you are sure that your client is able to listen effectively, the following facts need to be presented. Always back up verbal information with written material that the client can consult later and show to others.

Essential information

(a) The significance of being AB+ (that is, not having AIDS but being infectious to others).
(b) Routes of transmission – blood to blood and body fluids to blood.
(c) For women – the importance of not becoming pregnant.
(d) The limits of risk to others (no need to isolate yourself, have separate crockery, cutlery, towels, etc.).
(e) Safer sex practices.
(f) What to look for in terms of ill-health (persistent shortness of breath, dry irritating cough and fever, chest pains, difficulty in swallowing, severe and persistent diarrhoea, marked weight loss, changes in personality, unexplained skin lesions). Try to aim for a balance between denial/avoidance (taking no care at all) and obsession (worrying over every spot or sniffle). Many symptoms of AIDS (weight loss, night sweats, diarrhoea) can be produced by anxiety.
(g) Health boosting – nutrition, exercise, sleep, cutting down on alcohol, nicotine, and other drugs, keeping a positive attitude.

Who to tell

Encourage clients to discuss fully with you the implications of telling other people that they are AB+ before doing so. Support them in being responsible, but point out the limits of responsibility – that is, who needs to know for their own protection. Offer support in telling significant others, and counselling for them.

End of session

Assure clients of your availability – let them know when and where they can contact you and who to ask for in a crisis if you are not there. Make another appointment 'to see how you're getting on'. Get the message across that you don't expect them to get it all right immediately – especially changing to safer sex – or they may be afraid to tell you their difficulties. Provide clear written material as a back up. There is too much to remember without it.

Kubler-Ross (1969) has identified five stages of coping mechanisms that people pass through when they are faced with tragic news. Being identified as AB+ is, to all intents and purposes, being told that you have an incurable, terminal illness. It is useful to bear these stages in mind when counselling people who are AB+ and be aware of the dangers of them getting stuck in one stage. They are briefly reviewed below:

1. *Denial.* This can be an essential buffer against the shock of knowing. It is often manifested in questioning the test result. The danger of staying in this stage is that people will not be taking care of themselves or others if they do not accept their antibody status.

2. *Anger.* When the first stage of denial can no longer be maintained, it is replaced by rage – 'why me?' This is difficult for counsellors to cope with as it is often displaced on to them, so try not to take it personally. Wouldn't you be angry too? At the same time, clients need to be helped through this stage or they will alienate their family and friends, and become very lonely and isolated.

3. *Bargaining.* Really an attempt to postpone acceptance, and often associated with guilt.

4. *Depression.* This is really grief – for impending loss – and should be facilitated by the counsellor. Reassurance and cheerful opinion is not always appropriate and is usually an expression of the counsellor's own needs. If the sadness is repressed, then the client will not be able to move on to the next stage.

5. *Acceptance.* If the previous stages can be worked through, positive antibody status can be accepted and this can act as a catalyst for a safer, healthier life-style with more feeling of control and self-confidence.

The working environment

Agencies working with drug abusers need to be aware of their own working environment. All the precautions that we spell out in this section should always have been carried out anyway to avoid the spread of hepatitis B. Hepatitis B is much more virulent and easier to transmit than HIV, and it has been with us in drug agencies for years, yet we have taken very few precautions to combat its spread.

We have been working in a residential setting with HIV positive people now for three years. We have developed very strong and clear guidelines. These are centred on the assumption that everyone in our unit, resident, prospective client, and staff alike, must assume that they are AB+ and must take necessary precautions. These are quite simple. If anyone cuts themselves they must clean up any spilt blood themselves with a solution of nine parts water, one part bleach. Any open cuts must be dressed with sticky plaster or a bandage, and minor cuts needing dressing should be done by the individual him- or herself. Any more major damage necessitating someone else dressing the wound means that they should wear disposable gloves to do so. If any blood or other body fluid is spilled on clothes they should be washed in a hot wash (over 60 degrees). There should be no sharing of razors or toothbrushes and female residents and staff should be careful when disposing of menstrual products.

There should be very clear and concise education programmes for staff, residents, and clients, in day centres and agencies raising general health awareness, and also covering areas of needle-sharing practices, safer sex practices, and family contact. If everyone in an organisation considers themselves positive, then there will be very little chance of anyone in the working environment picking up HIV.

And remember –

YOU ARE MORE DANGEROUS TO PEOPLE WHO ARE HIV POSITIVE THAN THEY ARE TO YOU

If you go into work with a cold, flu or other infection and meet a client who is HIV positive, you may pass on your infection to them. What was a mild infection to you could result in someone with a compromised immune system developing a complex series of infections which could lead to death. It is a very important point to remember in your relationship with people who are HIV positive that it is in fact you who are the danger to them, and not the reverse.

This is reinforced by recent information on HIV infection in health care workers (Anon 1987c).

On 22 May 1987 the Center for Disease Control (CDC), Atlanta, reported three cases which appear to fulfil the criteria for occupationally-acquired HIV infection. These were three health care workers who were splashed on the skin in 1986, one of whom was also splashed in the mouth, with blood from patients infected with HIV. At interview none had alternative risk factors to explain their infections, but unrecognised or forgotten needle-stick exposures cannot be excluded:

1. A female with ungloved chapped hands, whose finger was in contact with blood for about 20 minutes while she assisted in the insertion of an arterial catheter at a cardiac arrest, developed fever, weight loss, and generalised lymphadenopathy, 21 days later. Blood collected eight months previously was HIV antibody negative but 16 weeks after the incident was HIV antibody positive.
2. A female phlebotomist with acne was splashed on the face and in the mouth while collecting blood in a vacuum container from an infected patient; she was wearing gloves at the time and washed the blood off immediately. Her blood was HIV antibody negative next day and eight weeks after the incident, but was positive nine months later. During the interim she sustained a scratch from a needle used to collect blood from an IV drug abuser of unknown serological status.
3. A female medical technologist spilled contaminated blood on the intact skin of her hands while manipulating a plasmapheresis machine. She was not wearing gloves and although she quickly washed off the blood, she might have touched an area of dermatitis on her ear. After five days her blood was HIV antibody negative, but eight weeks later she became febrile and developed a red, macular rash. Three months after the incident her blood was HIV antibody positive.

Similar cases were reported in a housewife who provided home nursing care to a man with AIDS, and a woman who looked after her infected son. Apart from these five cases there have been four authenticated accounts of occupationally-acquired HIV infection. All were female nurses who received accidental needle-stick inoculation injuries.

Although the degree of risk of transmission of HIV from exposures involving needle-stick injuries or blood splashes cannot be precisely defined, results of recent studies conducted at CDC (1097 exposures, one seroconversion), the National Institutes of Health (322 exposures, nil seroconversions), the University of California (63 exposures, nil seroconversions) and the Centre for Disease Surveillance and Control (CDSC) (150 exposures, nil seroconversions) suggest that this is extremely low. Health care workers can minimise the risk of exposure by following routinely recommended precautions when in contact with secretions from patients known to be infected with HIV, wearing gloves and washing the skin quickly after contamination with patients' body fluids, and by maintaining sensible standards of hygiene at all times.

The future

Over the next five years, drug agencies will have to learn to live with an increasing number of clients who are AB+. It is the responsibility of anyone working with drug users to ensure that their agency has a humane, well-formulated, and well-documented policy on HIV/AIDS, and that any agency to which they refer clients also has such a policy. This is by no means universal practice, and yet the next phase of the AIDS epidemic is on the horizon – drug users suffering from persistent generalised lymphadenopathy (PGL), AIDS-related complex (ARC) and the full AIDS syndrome in our treatment programmes and coming to our street agencies for help. There is a pressing need for comprehensive training and increased funding to meet the needs of our client groups in the future.

The expansion and support of existing facilities may be the way to ensure adequate provision for those AB+ drug users who want to stop. But what of those who don't – and are AB+ already or running the risk of infection at any time?

Over the last 15 years the emphasis in this country has been on abstinence, rehabilitation, and punitive measures against those who 'fail'. The AIDS crisis has highlighted the need, previously largely ignored, for damage limitation. We need to accept the necessity for the prescription of opiate substitutes or even of the opiates themselves so that this large group of people who are potentially at risk of infection can be reached with information and education. Then we can work with them – not exclusively towards a drug-free life, but towards a safer, healthier life with the aim of reducing needle sharing, the use of cut street drugs, and the whole criminal sub-culture that drives the drug users further underground.

As this chapter goes to press, the government has published its response to the Advisory Council's report on AIDS and Drug Misuse (1988). The Advisory Council made forty-seven recommendations, but only a few are singled out for any comment. The government declined to expand the needle-exchange schemes, to make any changes in policy on the treatment of drug users in prison, or to make any additional resources available to help prevent the spread of HIV infection amongst and from drug users. The main emphasis was on prevention of drug use through tough law enforcement and education – 'It is self-evident that if people do not start using drugs in the first place then they do not put themselves at risk of infection through this route'.

The government's response was immediately challenged by the Standing Conference on Drug Abuse in a press release dated 29 March 1988:

> The real challenge for the Government is whether they will step beyond the cosmetics of advertising, give real leadership and put resources into reaching the massive population of drug users who care little for fine words and want tangible help.

Many professionals already perceive drug takers as imposing a burden on over-stretched facilities. Compound that with the medical problems associated with ARC and AIDS and the need for specialist services for this group should be obvious. Where are those services, and when will they be available for the people who need them now?

References

Anon (1987a) 'More playing safe', *AIDS Letter*, 1 (1): 2.

Anon (1987b) 'Female to female transmission of HIV', *AIDS Letter*, 1 (4): 6.

Anon (1987c) 'Infection risks to health workers', *AIDS Letter*, 1 (2): 2.

Buning, E.C., Coutinho, R.A., Brussel, G.H.A. van, Santen, G.W. van, and Zadelhoff, A.W. van (1986) 'Preventing AIDS in drug addicts in Amsterdam', *The Lancet*, 1: 1435.

Carr, J. (1987) 'An injection of common sense', *The Nursing Times*, 83 (24): 19–20.

Department of Health and Social Security (1985), 'Introduction of a test for HTLV III antibody', CMO(85), 12.

Department of Health and Social Security (1988), 'Services for drug misusers – curbing the spread of AIDS and HIV infection', HC(88), 26.

Ghodse, A.H., Tregenza, G., and Li, M. (1987) 'Effect of fear of AIDS on sharing of injection equipment among drug abusers', *British Medical Journal*, 295: 698–9.

Kubler-Ross, E. (1969) *On death and dying*, London: Tavistock.

Marks, J. and Parry, A. (1987) 'Syringe exchange programmes for drug addicts', *The Lancet*, 1: 691–2.

Martin, P. (1986) 'New directions in residential care', Churchill Fellowship Report (unpublished).

Robertson, J.R., Skidmore, C.A., and Roberts, J.J.K. (1988) 'HIV infection in intravenous drug users: A follow-up study indicating changes in risk-taking behaviour', *British Journal of Addiction*, 83: 387–91.

Scottish Home and Health Department (1986) *Scottish Committee on HIV infection and intravenous drug misuse*, Edinburgh.

Strang, J., Heathcote, S., and Watson, P. (1987) 'Habit moderation in injecting drug addicts', *Health Trends*, 19: 16–18.

Part Three

Developments in Services

Chapter Nine

Drug treatment and prescribing practice: what can be learned from the past?

Jenny Wilks

In recent years, in response to an increase in awareness of the extent of problem drug use, there has been an expansion of services and a range of new approaches to treatment, largely influenced by the *Treatment and Rehabilitation* report of the Advisory Council on the Misuse of Drugs (1982). However, this was not accompanied by a great deal of debate about the general philosophy underlying services for drug users, and there is arguably insufficient clarity or agreement on what assumptions are operating in different agencies. In the past year (partly in response to the AIDS threat) there has been a revival of the debate around prescribing practices, which indicates both how difficult it is to reach agreement and the need for a re-think of treatment policies. The aim of this chapter is to explore the assumptions underlying drug services and the implications of these for treatment policies, looking in particular at what past experiences suggest for future directions in drug treatment. The focus will be on illicit drug use, particularly heroin, but many of the issues are relevant to wider aspects of drug services.

Models of Treatment

The basic question of why to treat problem drug use at all could be answered in several different ways, each of which has different implications for the kind of treatment that would be offered. Treatment can be seen as a logical consequence of any of several premises, for example:

Abstinence-oriented model

Drug users should be offered medical and psychological help with the aim of achieving a drug-free life.

Harm-reduction model

Treatment should aim to reduce the legal, social, and health problems caused *to the user* by drug use, and hence improve their quality of life and perhaps prolong life.

Social control model

Treatment can reduce the problem caused *to society* by drug users, and is therefore necessary to contain these effects, that is, to control illicit drug use and related crime.

The drawing of sharp distinctions between these models is somewhat artificial, and many workers would argue that their services are to varying degrees informed by all these models and more. This might seem to be ideal, since it implies a flexible response based on the needs of individual clients. The problem is that these premises have certain logical corollaries which are mutually incompatible, for example:

Abstinence model

Treatment services have nothing to offer to drug users who are unwilling (or unable) to give up drugs.

Harm-reduction model

Treatment services aim to minimise the dangers of drug use; reduction/cessation of drug use is one way to achieve this but there are other strategies which are more appropriate in many cases.

Social control model

Treatment services' policies are based on what impact they will have on people *outside* the treatment setting, regardless of what effect this has on the users in treatment.

In many clinical situations these models would therefore lead to different responses, for example, in deciding what to offer to a heroin user who wants a prescription but is not willing to attempt withdrawal at present. The abstinence model would lead to an attempt to increase motivation and persuade the person to accept detoxification and perhaps residential treatment in view of the perceived difficulty of sustaining a drug-free state. The harm-reduction model might offer an extended prescription as part of an attempt to facilitate safer drug use. The social control model might also lead to open-ended prescribing, but this would be contingent on evidence that the person is not supplementing this illegally or committing other crimes.

Treatment agencies are rarely very explicit about which premise(s) they are founded upon, and tend to operate (and to be under pressure from outside to operate) with a contradictory mix of all three. For example, staff may argue fervently that they are aiming to help users (whether they define this as 'cure' or 'harm reduction') and that they are not in the business of social control, but may be under pressure from legal agencies to show that their work has an impact on the illicit drug scene and related crime.

Whatever happened to the British system?

Although the drug scene has been continually changing over the last couple of decades, any discussion of the effects of different policies and philosophies on drug users, drug workers, and society needs to be set in the context of the historical development of drug services in the UK. Before the 1920s anyone could buy various preparations of opium from a chemist, and opiates were probably more widely used in Victorian times than at any time since. When this practice became illegal, the so-called 'British system' came into being, under the recommendation of the Rolleston Committee, whereby any doctor could prescribe any drug (including heroin and cocaine) to treat addiction to the drug. This could include long-term maintenance prescribing, where attempts at withdrawal had failed and where the individual could lead a stable life-style if they had a steady dose of the drug. There were very few people dependent on these drugs, and all were of therapeutic (that is, iatrogenic) or professional origin. For nearly forty years this situation did not seem to change, and treatment was based on a medical (though not abstinence-oriented) model, aimed at the individual addicts, while also having a social control purpose in preventing these drug users from creating a demand for an illicit market.

The late 1950s and early 1960s saw an increase in both the number and types of drug users. Most were by then young recreational users who were supplied by a black market fed by surplus NHS-prescribed heroin (particularly from a small number of doctors who vastly over-prescribed). The precise reasons for these changes are unclear, but the policy which had permitted doctors to prescribe heroin and cocaine to addicts was perceived as a major contributor to the problem. However, it was still believed that availability of heroin from legal sources kept black market prices to a minimum, and prevented illegal importation and sale from becoming lucrative enough for organised crime to get involved. The present-day reader may be tempted to dismiss this as very naïve, but it should be borne in mind that in the 1960s there was very little evidence of imported heroin being sold in the UK.

Social control and the clinics

When the original Drug Dependence clinics were set up in 1968, under the recommendations of the second Brain Committee, one of the main objectives was to contain the spread of heroin addiction. Along with the assumption that legal availability of heroin would undercut the black market went the recognition that clinic prescriptions could themselves feed this market. Clinics were therefore expected to strike a balance between prescribing sufficient opiates so that people would not need to supplement them by buying illicit heroin, but not so much that they would sell any surplus. The clinics thus aimed to control both the supply and demand sides of the black market. This rather daunting task does not seem to have much to do with treatment or therapeutic goals, and it is questionable whether it should be part of the function of a clinic to maintain the exact balance, even if one exists. At the same time it is an inescapable, if unpalatable, aspect of treatment that whatever happens in the clinics has repercussions on the wider drug scene.

The abstinence model and the clinics

While accepting maintenance, the Brain Committee emphasised that the long-term goal was withdrawal for most addicts. It was assumed that a drug taker who was not initially motivated to withdraw might, through the building of therapeutic relationships with staff, gradually become so. (Critics pointed out that by being so supportive and by prescribing, the clinics may in fact be helping people to sustain their existing life-style and preventing them from having a compelling incentive to try to stop using (Edwards 1969).) Quite apart from social control considerations, this dual agenda meant that even within treatment objectives there was considerable ambiguity over whether the clinics' main role was to help highly-motivated people to come off, or to prescribe to anyone with an opiate habit so that the drug user could avoid the black market and the health risks of illicit drugs, and also ideally over a period of time be encouraged to decide to withdraw. While both these aims can be seen as abstinence-oriented, they are clearly different in their implications for treatment policy and practice.

Harm reduction and the clinics

Whatever the official function of the clinics, at first they did at least serve the purpose of keeping contact with 'the street'; for the first few years relatively few heroin addicts were not in contact with a clinic, at least on and off, and therefore most users had at least some access to medical care. (By the late 1970s, the majority of new Home Office notifications were from outside clinics.) In practice, therefore, the clinics' role may have been one of harm reduction, in so far as they gave their clients access to uncut, pharmaceutical opiates, sterile needles and syringes, and a break from the illicit drug scene. Evidence as to whether this did, in fact, reduce harm is mixed; for example, there was still a considerable amount of needle sharing, although there is some evidence of a higher incidence of non-sterile injecting, physical complications, and mortality among heroin users who were not on a prescription (Paxton *et al.* 1978).

However, harm reduction was not the official role of the clinics; so whether or not they were achieving some success at it, they were in any case being judged by other criteria. From outside they were assessed from the perspective of social control, while from the inside a treatment model was stressed. Eventually they were viewed as failing on both counts.

The conflict of treatment and social control

The attempt to reconcile these two models led early on to two major sources of dissatisfaction among clinic staff. From the social control point of view it appeared that, even after the clinics were set up, the prescriptions (which initially were relatively generous, people usually being given what they had been receiving before from non-clinic doctors) continued to contribute to the black market. Illicitly sold heroin was still largely of NHS origin, so the clinics were seen to be failing on the supply side of controlling illicit drug use, even though they may have been temporarily instrumental in minimising the demand for an alternative (that is, illegally manufactured and imported) source of illicit heroin.

From the treatment point of view there was much frustration among staff, who saw themselves as care-givers, not as 'policemen in white coats' (Stimson 1978), and realised that what is sensible from the point of view of social control may not be so from the point of view of treatment and vice versa. From the point of view of controlling the drug problem (by attracting people to the clinic and providing licit drugs), a maintenance prescribing policy might be preferred, but it conflicts with therapeutic ideals since people are not reducing their drug dependence. The fact that the clinics were expected to reduce the availability of illicit heroin also introduced into the staff/patient relationship an atmosphere of conflict and coercion, since the control of individual patients was the only mechanism by which the clinics could attempt to control the wider drug problem. This militated against mutual agreement on goals between staff and patients; bargaining about the dose became a common feature, and changes in the dose or the drug given could even be used as a disciplinary measure, so that the status of the 'script' was raised out of proportion to the role it might otherwise have played. In response to these issues clinic policies and approaches gradually changed in ways which attempted to focus more strongly on the treatment aspect, and also to increase control on the supply side of the illicit market.

The evolution of clinic policies

The 1970s witnessed three shifts in prescribing policy: from prescription of heroin to methadone, injectable to oral drugs, and maintenance to time-limited withdrawal. The reasons for these changes are complex. Methadone has the advantage of only requiring one dose daily, and is therefore more suitable for encouraging clients to stabilise their working and social lives. This would imply that it is particularly suitable for long-term maintenance, but it is almost invariably used in short-term withdrawal programmes too. There are obvious medical reasons for preferring the oral to the intravenous route of administration, however these reasons (with the exception of HIV) applied in the 1960s as well, but the move away from prescribing has been particularly marked since the mid-1970s (Woodcock 1984).

The concept of 'stabilisation' via maintenance prescriptions was virtually abandoned during the 1970s, at least for new patients, and has come to have a very secondary role, relative to withdrawal and rehabilitation. It had been based on the middle-aged therapeutic and professional addicts of the past, who led conventional lives as long as they were on a prescription. By the 1960s this was changing; most new addicts were young people who had lived more socially unconventional lives with or without drugs, and there is some evidence that a maintenance prescription was no longer a recipe for a 'normalisation' of life-style. Research at St. George's and St. Thomas' Hospitals in London between 1968 and 1975 (Weipert *et al.* 1978) found that, apart from continuity of treatment and decrease in drug-related hospital admissions, the only evidence of stabilisation was a slightly improved work record and there was no change in death rates or crime. Oppenheimer *et al.* (1979) found that the only addicts of 1969 in their sample who later achieved a very stable life-style were those who had managed to become abstinent. This supports the impression of clinics that younger, recreational users tend not to develop a stable life-style even when they are on an opiate prescription. They are therefore pushed more toward withdrawal, although the logic of this is somewhat questionable, since if these people cannot bring some order into their lives when on a prescription they might be even less likely to when not on one.

The other premise behind the setting up of the clinics which has lost favour is the idea that it is possible to undercut the black market by legal prescription. Early arguments that the 'British system' had been successful in doing this seem to have been premature; but this begs the question of whether the whole system was misguided, or whether the way it was implemented and modified prevented it from achieving these aims. A major dilemma for clinic staff is that while they may justifiably feel that it is not their job to influence the activities of the criminal and drug-dealing underworld, they also recognise that a therapeutic policy cannot be pursued independently of the problem on 'the street'.

To assess current practice and decide future policies, it is useful to look at the evidence, such as exists, for what impact the clinics seem to have had on both their clients and the wider drug scene.

Impact on clients

Long-term studies give a picture of what happened to heroin addicts who attended the clinics during the first ten years; however, causal relationships are very difficult to establish. Stimson and Oppenheimer (1984) found that, ten years on, nearly 40 per cent had successfully become abstinent. It is not clear what, if anything, this had to do with treatment (it is possible that they would have stopped using anyway, and that long-term prescriptions may even have prolonged their addiction), but it is a more optimistic outcome than might have been expected. A similar number (38 per cent) were still attending and on prescriptions. The authors point out that the interpretation of the latter figure depends on what one expects from treatment: that it should supply a cure from addiction, or help addicts lead a reasonably stable life on drugs; although, as stated above, a long-term prescription did not necessarily go hand in hand with a stable life-style, many of the latter group evidenced few problems outside their opiate dependence. This points to one of the major hurdles in achieving a broad agreement on drug treatment policy, since one's assumptions about the aims of treatment will not only affect what kind of treatment is offered, but how outcome results are evaluated.

Another very relevant study in view of the gradual changes in clinic policy was conducted between 1972 and 1976 by Hartnoll *et al.* (1980) and involved randomly assigning people to either injectable heroin or oral methadone prescriptions. Twelve months after entering treatment, the heroin group were more likely to have continued in treatment; the methadone group had a higher drop-out rate *but* were more likely to have discontinued regular opiate use. This study was, at the time, widely believed to show little difference between heroin and oral methadone, and was therefore used as justification for preferring the latter, that is, as providing a scientific rationale for an already occurring policy change. The findings are clearly more complex, and indicate that either option involves a 'trade off', so that which option will be preferred depends on treatment aims and philosophy. A considerably higher abstinence rate was achieved by prescribing oral methadone, but at the expense of a higher arrest rate and greater use of illicit drugs among those who did not become abstinent. Prescribing heroin tended to maintain the 'status quo', whereas those prescribed oral methadone tended to polarise into more extreme outcomes (for better or worse) on a number of measures of drug involvement and social stability. Rather than vindicating one or other approach, the results suggest that it may be impossible for clinics to find a policy that would both result in an optimal number achieving abstinence and also permit long-term contact with a high number of users in order to ameliorate their illicit drug use and related problems. Oral methadone may be more 'therapeutic' in terms of discouraging continued drug use, but it leaves a group of heavily drug-involved people outside contact with clinics; this has implications at both social control and harm-reduction levels.

Impact on the drug scene

In retrospect, changes can be seen to have occurred 'on the street' during the first decade of the clinics, but again causal relationships are very unclear. Initially, the clinics may not have been entirely unsuccessful in restricting the availability of heroin, since the number of notifications to the Home Office levelled off in 1969 and 1970. Seizures of black market heroin at that time were almost exclusively of pharmaceutical origin, indicating that the NHS was still the major source of supply of illicit heroin. By 1971, already less than a quarter of those on prescriptions were getting any heroin from the clinics (Woodcock 1984). It was at about this time that police and customs began to seize the first significant quantities of illicitly manufactured heroin intended for the UK market (rising from 1.1 kg in 1971 to 366 kg in 1985). In the 1970s, during which years the clinics tightened up, the black market continued to flourish but became more and more dependent on imported heroin. Clinics were therefore now failing to control on the demand side, but by this time the prevailing view was that it was impossible for them to do so and the aim was at least to reduce the NHS-supplied part of the black market to a minimum.

The increase in illicitly manufactured heroin is at least consistent with the view that the clinics, in the attempt to avoid supplying the black market, went too far the other way and erred on the side of too restrictive prescribing. It is important to note that this does not mean that, in the very different situation of the late 1980s, an increasing liberalisation of opiate prescribing would necessarily have any significant impact on the extent of the illicit market. However, now that there is a relatively reliable black market in heroin, and very little (particularly for new patients) at the clinics, there is less incentive to enter treatment; harm reduction can therefore be offered to a smaller proportion of users via this setting.

The context of new directions in the 1980s

Twenty years on from the inception of the clinics, the drug scene has changed dramatically. The illicit market is very different (pharmaceutical heroin being so rare that some users have called it the 'champagne of the opiates'); there is a new mode of heroin use by smoking, which was very rare pre-1979; there has been a large rise in the number of notifications as well as evidence of a continuing increase in the use of other drugs; and there is a new and unprecedented health threat posed by AIDS. These developments necessitate much careful consideration in developing future directions in drug treatment practice, using the experience of the last twenty years as a guide while recognising the changes that have occurred. The AIDS threat demands rapid responses, but it is vital that changes in practice are thought through and not hastily adopted in an effort to be seen to be doing something.

The following are some aspects of the current context of drug treatment which decisions about philosophy and direction need to take into account, some of which are new to the 1980s and some of which have always been relevant.

What do drug users want from treatment?

The task of drugs agencies would be easier if there were agreement between staff and clients about goals and methods of treatment. However in clinics there is frequently a 'clash of perspectives about the nature and meaning of drug use, the purpose of the clinic, rights to a prescription and the purpose of therapy' (Stimson 1978). For most clients the reason for attending the clinic, at least in the first instance, is to receive an NHS prescription for opiates. However, from the clinic's point of view, drug users are accepted for treatment on the assumption that they want to try to stop using. This leads to a greater implicit selection of clients than in the 1960s, when the goal of abstinence was seen more as a longer-term ideal than a short-term aim, so that fewer drug takers connect with the treatment on offer, and those who do come may find it difficult to be completely honest about what they would really like from the clinic. This is not conducive to progress toward either risk reduction or control of drug use, which requires a joint effort with mutual trust and respect between staff and clients. This is not to suggest that drug users should be given whatever they demand from services, but that more effort needs to be made to involve them in decision-making about service development and the choice of treatment interventions available.

Range of treatments on offer

Although there is now a wider range of treatment agencies (both statutory and non-statutory) offering a greater choice to the potential client, within the clinics and other medical settings the range of options has narrowed in recent years. Most clinics now adopt more structured treatment contracts where the prescription is only part of the 'package' and often the period/schedule of reduction is agreed in advance. This has two effects:

1. In practice there is a more consistent 'British system' than there was in the 1960s, with a rather stereotyped treatment response offered to all heroin users regardless of individual differences.
2. However, perhaps mitigating the above, there is much inconsistency between theory and practice, and ensuing frustration among staff.

Ghodse (1983), describing the use of time-limited detoxification contracts, states: 'There is obviously a risk of relapse and repeated contracts may be necessary.' This raises the question of what is the distinction between repetition of time-limited contracts and long-term or maintenance prescribing.

Range of drugs used

Clinics were set up in response to a rise in heroin use in the 1960s, and this has tended to remain the chief focus of most. In the late 1970s in particular this was not relevant to most drug users, who used a variety of drugs, especially barbiturates and amphetamines. The last few years have seen a rise in heroin use, apparently as a result of the fashion for 'chasing the dragon', so the focus of clinics on opiates might appear more justified; but most clinics still see older, injecting users, not the younger users who are represented in the increased notifications, and there is still very little, if anything, offered to users of other drugs. This is now of particular concern because many people use non-opiates (for example, amphetamines and cocaine) intravenously; if they do not find agencies accessible to them they will not be reached by risk-reduction information around AIDS/HIV.

Impact of treatment policies on 'the street'

The experience of 1980 onwards seems to have finally laid to rest the idea that treatment services can contain the wider drug problem. The huge influx of imported heroin and the introduction of smoking it, combined with various social factors (for example, the rise in long-term unemployment among young people), has rendered the clinics relatively helpless to make an impact on the wider problem, and thus tended to reinforce their retreat from the notion that they are involved in social control. However, critics argue that clinics are now acting as if they can ignore the wider setting completely and may be facilitating the continuing increase in the black market: 'There is a relationship between what a doctor does with the prescription pad . . . and what happens to the broader problem' (Spear 1986).

Public health policy around AIDS/HIV

Current debate about the future of drug treatment services is inevitably coloured by the context of a government which, since the beginning of the 1980s, has aimed to reduce state support for health and welfare services, and to increase the emphasis on law and order. This has led to more punitive approaches to the drug problem, and an emphasis on control via police and customs, rather than clinics and other drugs agencies. The concept of decriminalising or increasing access to any drugs to curb the black market is hardly open to serious debate in such an atmosphere. Similarly, any shift in emphasis from prevention of all drug use to prevention of particularly disfunctional or dangerous drug use is seen as condoning or even encouraging drug use. The great danger of such totally prohibitive attitudes is that they inhibit the teaching of less risky modes of drug use.

However, this attitude is beginning to change, with the recognition that any new moves and directions in the field of drug treatment must at every point take into account the threat of HIV infection to the drug-injecting population, and via them to other people. Making syringes and needles available along with good health education is one fundamental harm-reduction strategy which has achieved some acceptability, largely because drug users, as a so-called 'bridging group', pose a threat to the general population. While anyone working in the drugs field must welcome any moves to make syringes widely available, this may be less likely to succeed if it is done in isolation rather than being part of a comprehensive attempt at health education and risk reduction among drug takers. Injecting drug users have always been at risk of illnesses caused by unsterile needles (for example, hepatitis, septicaemia and gangrene), but the supply of needles has never previously been given the serious attention that it is now getting, and advice on how to use other drugs more safely still attracts strong criticism (Corina 1987). It is arguable that if harm reduction had always been at the forefront of drugs policies, syringes would have been more widely available in the past, and the rate of HIV infection among drug users might have been much lower now.

The AIDS threat highlights the ethics and politics of harm reduction, and although a major re-think of treatment policies was overdue even without AIDS, it makes this particularly urgent. Any changes in policy must be made with consideration, not only of the impact on drug users in treatment and on 'the street', but also on the spread of the virus. Drugs workers also need to anticipate that this issue could lead to a new twist in the conflict between treatment and social control, and that drugs agencies may find demands being made on them to protect society from HIV via their treatment policies, in ways which may be difficult to reconcile with therapeutic aims. In the current political climate, repressive measures against AIDS are quite probable, even though they would be very dangerous from the point of view of public health.

The prescribing debate

Due to a combination of increasing concern about the implications of AIDS/HIV for the treatment of drug takers, and increasing polarisation of attitudes and treatment policies between the Drug Dependence Clinics and private doctors in addiction, the past year has witnessed a renewal of the debate about appropriate prescribing. However, although this debate tends to focus on the currently fashionable concept of 'flexible prescribing', it has frequently been characterised by the adoption of rather inflexible and extreme positions.

On the one hand is the view, expressed by Marks (1987) and some private doctors (Dally 1987), that maintenance prescribing (including prescribing injectable heroin) is an appropriate way of protecting drug takers from the various legal and health consequences of drug use (including HIV) until such time as they are ready to withdraw. Arguments in favour of this perspective are frequently passionate and emotive but make surprisingly sparse reference to the experience of the late 1960s when a maintenance policy prevailed. Past experience indicates that maintenance prescribing *per se* is not sufficient to ensure harm minimisation or social control of the drug problem, and there is a need for further study of what additional components are needed in the total treatment 'package' if long-term prescribing is to be effective in reducing health-damaging and illicit drug use.

At the other extreme there is a view that coming off heroin is the least difficult part of treatment, and that the main thrust of the therapeutic endeavour should be, after a relatively brief withdrawal, to support people in remaining drug free. The fact that controlled detoxification can be done relatively painlessly, yet many users repeatedly relapse even after considerable periods drug free, would seem to support this view, and it has stimulated the development of treatment packages under the general heading of 'relapse prevention' (Marlatt and George 1984). The high rate of relapse suggests that, while interventions aimed at facilitating abstinence and reducing relapse are certainly needed, there may be little to be gained by encouraging people to try to come off drugs before they are ready to do so; the dilemma is whether they should therefore be offered long-term prescriptions in the meantime, or left to fend for themselves on 'the street'. In Stimson and Oppenheimer's (1984) sample, three-quarters of the forty subjects who had become abstinent had been withdrawn by their clinic, but only after an average of four years on a prescription. After withdrawal they had received little therapeutic support, maintaining abstinence on their own. The contribution of treatment to their progress is hard to judge, but the pattern is interesting in view of current moves to offer faster withdrawal, and emphasis on follow-up support to help people stay off drugs, since this group seems to have done it the other way round as far as treatment is concerned.

The term 'flexible prescribing' has not yet been adequately defined, but would seem to imply first, individually-tailored treatment responses based on assessment of each client's needs and abilities, particularly the extent to which they are currently able or willing to control their drug use; second, acceptance that short-term detoxification contracts may fail repeatedly and may need replacing with a longer-term prescription; and third, an approach to extended prescriptions in which their appropriateness would be periodically reassessed so that withdrawal might be attempted more frequently than the term 'maintenance' implies. In relation to the issue of HIV, there is also increasing awareness that, as more clinic clients become HIV-positive and show symptoms of AIDS/ARC, the continued injection of 'street' drugs (and the stress involved in attempting to withdraw) may be immunosuppressive, and a stable prescription, while not ideal, may be the preferred option in many cases. This is not to suggest that drug users with HIV should not be offered as much support and encouragement as anyone else in attempting to achieve abstinence; but rather that their HIV-status is a factor to take into account in deciding treatment responses if they are unable or unwilling to come off drugs.

It is unfortunate that the term 'flexible prescribing' seems to have rapidly come to be associated with 'maintenance prescribing', since any one approach to prescribing (whether maintenance or withdrawal) cannot, by definition, be very flexible. However, it is probably inevitable that a move from current clinic policies toward a more flexible approach would increase the number and length of extended prescriptions offered, and this has a number of implications which require consideration and evaluation.

As discussed above, one of the difficulties in attempting to assess the impact of relatively liberal prescribing (both on harm reduction and social control) is that, while both clinic policies and the illicit drug scene went through a series of changes during the 1970s, there was insufficient attempt at that time to assess the extent to which one was a function of the other, and it is very difficult to assess causal relationships retrospectively. Indeed, the available evidence of changing trends in the clinics and on 'the street' could be used quite plausibly to support either argument: that the illicit heroin market flourished because the clinics tightened up, or that the clinics tightened up because the illicit market was growing regardless. If 'flexible prescribing' is to include an increase in the number of people on long-term prescriptions, it is vital that this is done with considered planning of the criteria for such prescriptions, as well as close monitoring of how each new development in clinical practice is reflected in the effects of treatment (on drug use and on the spread of HIV), and in evidence of what is happening on 'the street'.

It is also important to reassess the notion of 'stabilisation' of the drug-taker's life-style: what it means, under what circumstances does it occur, and to what extent? This needs to be defined realistically; there is little point in including 'legal employment' as a criterion of a stable life-style when so many clients have little access to this regardless of their drug use. At a minimum, however, most clinics would want to see evidence that the person's drug use had become stable. This raises the issue of what sanctions to apply when people supplement their prescriptions with illicit drugs, which opens up the area of possible conflicts between treatment/harm reduction and social control. In order to attract the highest number of heroin-dependent people into treatment, where they can be offered some protection from health risks, prescribing heroin might be best, since methadone is generally seen by drug takers as a poor substitute. However, if methadone is prescribed, it is easier to monitor (by urinanalysis) the general extent to which people stick to their prescription, and to respond in some way (that is, by a change in therapeutic approach) if they do not. Similar conflicts pertain to the prescribing of oral or injectible opiates; if one of the criticisms of long-term prescribing is that it reinforces drug taking, the use of oral prescriptions might at least break one aspect of the person's habit as well as being preferable medically. However, it may again make illicit drug use more likely. A comprehensive harm-reduction policy demands that, even while on a prescription, users must have access to clean needles and syringes, even though it may appear illogical to prescribe oral methadone while also encouraging them to make use of the local needle exchange for equipment in which they can only inject 'street' drugs.

There are some wider practical and ethical problems associated with increasing liberalism in prescribing. There are so many more heroin users than in 1968 that if a significantly higher proportion of them were offered extended prescriptions this could become a disproportionate amount of an agency's workload. This would be likely to detract from the time and resources available for psychosocial therapy and support, which would militate against both successful withdrawal and abstinence for those who attempted it, and stabilisation of life-style for those who did not. Indeed, there is a risk that the whole flavour of the clinics could change back to a narrower medical model. In recent years there has been a considerable increase in the role of other professionals in drugs services; long-term prescribing could once again bring drug dependence far more under the exclusive domain of the medical profession. This could be to the detriment of overall care, with insufficient attention to the psychological and social aspects of clients' problems, particularly if doctors were so busy prescribing that they had insufficient time to utilise their own therapeutic skills.

Serious ethical issues are also raised by the possibility that, if clinics were perceived as much more liberal in their prescribing practices, many recently-addicted or non-regular users of heroin would present for prescriptions, and it can be difficult for clinics to differentiate these from users with long-term dependency. (This of course begs the question of whether there is ever a case for prescribing, on social control or harm-reduction grounds, to people who have been identified as non-dependent or irregular drug takers.) The serious risk of very liberal prescribing is that it could create a new generation of partly-iatrogenic chronic opiate addicts who will become the clinics' 'old-timers' of the 1990s, where in many cases they might otherwise have eventually achieved abstinence. While a stable prescription of pharmaceutical opiates might be agreed to be less harmful than chaotic use of street drugs, the medical support of an increased dependence on opiates than would otherwise have occurred can scarcely be called 'harm reduction'.

A major problem in relation to this is that many clients would, at least initially, prefer a long-term prescription. If this is too readily offered, they may not even attempt to withdraw and will not discover whether they could have achieved it. On the other hand, if clients know that long-term prescribing is not even an option, they may be more likely to resent the limited range of treatments on offer and 'rebel' by arguing about the prescription or not coming to treatment at all. If they feel that an extended prescription may be a future option if all else fails (that is, that they will not be rejected by the clinic if they repeatedly lapse), they may be more able and willing to work with their therapist on a collaborative effort of which the primary aim is to bring drug use under complete control, but which recognises that initial treatment plans may later require revision. Similarly, treatment can be abstinence-oriented but still relatively long term, perhaps initially working toward intermediate goals short of abstinence (Strang 1987).

The foregoing discussion has posed more questions than suggested answers to the prescribing debate. However, it is clear that it is premature and destructive to take up polarising positions on the issue and that the drug scene in the 1980s is so different from that in the past that any new shifts in policy must be monitored and assessed in terms of their impact on the current problem. Any particular policy may now have a quite different effect on clients and on the heroin problem than it had, or would have had, in the 1960s and 1970s.

Conclusion

The next few years are likely to see considerable changes in the drug scene and in drug services, as agencies (and government departments) work out their responses to issues such as harm reduction, prescribing, and AIDS/HIV, particularly in the light of the recommendations of the Advisory Council on the Misuse of Drugs report (1988) on the latter. Debate and decision-making on these issues needs to take place with consideration not just of treatment practice, but also at the level of the 'models' underlying this, since (as described at the beginning of this chapter) different philosophies of treatment have different implications for clinical management. At a time of flux and controversy in the drugs field it is particularly important that agencies should be clear about the implicit assumptions under which they are operating, and that they consider whether their treatment methods and policies follow logically from these.

This does not mean that it is necessary, or even desirable, that every service should agree on treatment philosophy and practice, which would in any case be virtually impossible. Harm reduction among drug takers is not inconsistent with the provision of abstinence-oriented treatment facilities, so long as the drug taker has some choice over which aspect is emphasised for their particular treatment at that time, and so long as drug workers are not in conflict about which approach is the 'best' and see them instead as complementary or as different stages on a long-term process of change. The social control issue is more difficult, since this may sometimes conflict with what the client wants or needs at that time. All drugs agencies need to consider what impact, if any, the policies they pursue are likely to have on the wider drug scene, but they also need to reconcile the demands of society with the needs of their client group. Where external demands are made which are untenable for a treatment service, workers may need to resist being used as a mechanism for areas of influence which are not usually part of the remit of therapists and health care workers.

Past experience indicates that the long-term implications and effects of any major changes in drug services will not be immediately apparent. Perhaps the most important lesson to be learned from the past is therefore that new directions must be more closely monitored and evaluated, and should not become fossilised by premature dogmatism. Whatever treatment model, or hybrid of models, is preferred, any criteria for judging new directions in drug services should at least be guided by the principle of *nil nocere*: first, do no harm.

References

Ashton, M. (1981) *Theory and Practice in the New British System*, London: Institute for the Study of Drug Dependence.

Corina, A. (1987) 'The media press the panic button', *Mersey Drugs Journal*, 1 (2): 8–10.

Dally, A. (1987) 'Stabilise not criminalise', *Druglink*, 2 (1): 14.

Advisory Council on the Misuse of Drugs (1982) *Treatment and Rehabilitation*, London: HMSO.

Advisory Council on the Misuse of Drugs (1988) *AIDS and Drug Misuse, Part 1*, London: HMSO.

Edwards, G. (1969) 'The British approach to the treatment of heroin addiction', *The Lancet*, 12 April, pp. 768–72.

Ghodse, A.H. (1983) 'Treatment of drug addiction in London', *The Lancet*, 19 March, pp. 636–9.

Hartnoll, R.L., Mitcheson, M.C., Battersby, A., Brown, G., Ellis, M., Fleming, P., and Hedley, N. (1980) 'Evaluation of heroin maintenance in controlled trial', *Arch. Gen. Psychiatry*, 37: 877–84.

Marks, J. (1987) 'State rationed drugs', *Druglink*, 2 (4): 14.

Marlatt, A. and George, W.H. (1984) 'Relapse prevention: introduction and overview of the model', *British Journal of Addiction*, 79 (3): 261–73.

Oppenheimer, E., Stimson, G.V., and Thorley, A. (1979) 'Seven-year follow-up of heroin addicts: abstinence and continued use compared', *British Medical Journal*, 2: 627–30.

Paxton, R., Mullin, P., and Beattie, J. (1978) 'The effects of methadone maintenance with opioid takers', *Brit. J. Psychiat.*, 132: 473–81.

Phillipson, R.V. (1978) 'The British narcotics system', *Report series*, 13 (2), US National Institute on Drug Abuse: Rockville, Md.

Spear, B. (1986) quoted in Malyon, T., *New Statesman*, 17 October, pp. 7–10.

Stimson, G.V. (1978) 'Clinics: care or control?' *NewsRelease*, 5 (1): 14–16.

Stimson, G.V. and Oppenheimer, E. (1984) *Heroin Addiction*, London: Tavistock.

Strang, J. (1987) 'The prescribing debate', *Druglink* 2 (4): 10–11.

Weipert, G.D., Bewley, T.H., and d'Orban, P.T. (1978) 'Outcomes for 575 British opiate addicts entering treatment between 1968 and 1975', *Bulletin on Narcotics* 30 (1): 21–32.

Woodcock, J. (1984) *The Role of the Prescribing Clinic in the British Response to Drug Abuse*, London: Institute for the Study of Drug Dependence.

Chapter Ten

The Community Drug Team: current practice

Justine Schneider, Paul Davis,
Will Nuzum, and Gerald Bennett

In the middle years of the 1980s some of the new statutory services for problem drug takers started calling themselves Community Drug Teams (CDTs). This title reflected the similarity between their aspirations and those of other 'Community' Teams, particularly Community Alcohol Teams (CATs) which had developed during the previous few years. It is too early to provide a comprehensive description and evaluation of these services; this chapter looks at three very different examples in order to provide a snapshot of their organisation, philosophy, and operation.

CDTs are staffed mainly by members of statutory services providing a mix of professions, and employed by different agencies. They differ from the longer-established drug clinics by not being tied to a hospital, although some teams are based in hospitals. Their main task is to provide a direct service, although training and consultancy may also be important activities. They complement pre-existing services, such as prescribing clinics and advisory services, but are often the only specialist service for drug takers, and frequently act as a ginger group for developing better services. They also tend to take a wider view of the type of help drug takers may require, away from a narrow medical view of detoxification, that may encompass health, housing, employment, and leisure.

The background to CDTs

The experience of non-statutory organisations

During the 1960s and 1970s non-statutory services, particularly in London, set up day centres and street agencies, which presented alternatives and additions to the statutory services, and a focus away from the disease model and towards the individual's problems. Three major roles of street agencies are advocacy on behalf of drug users, direct counselling or advice to users and their families, and liaison with statutory agencies, for example, regarding health, housing, or probation. The work of these agencies shows the value of informal, accessible services which are easily approached and used and which are persistent in their availability. They are easy to approach and easy to return to.

Changing attitudes towards drug use and prescribing

Prescribing drugs to drug users is seen less and less as the most important component among services for drug users. This accompanied a loss of conviction that methadone provided a 'cure' for opiate addiction, and signalled the end of the psychiatrists' supposed monopoly in providing services. The second Brain Committee, in 1965, envisaged a multidisciplinary approach for the drug clinics, but this was not widely in operation. The Advisory Council on the Misuse of Drugs (ACMD), in its *Treatment and Rehabilitation* report of 1982, argued that:

> Although many of the problems related to drug misuse are personal and social as well as medical and legal, current treatment responses have been strongly influenced by the historical emphasis on opioids in drug legislation to the detriment of a naturally evolving and wider multidisciplinary treatment and rehabilitation service.

Prescribing continues to play an important part in drug services, but is increasingly seen as just one component, which can be provided by generic medical practitioners in the community, rather than just by hospital-based specialists. GPs were encouraged to participate more in prescribing for opiate users, with abstinence as the goal, as embodied in the *Guidelines of good clinical practice in the treatment of drug misusers* (DHSS 1984).

Changing patterns of drug taking

Drug-taking patterns changed significantly in Britain during the late 1970s and early 1980s. Heroin became cheaper, and its use more widespread, both geographically and between social classes. This led to a more diffuse approach to drug problems. They became a matter of concern for many statutory agencies, such as schools, youth services, probation and social services, in addition to mental health workers. Consequently drug policy became more politicised and central government began to play a leading role in formulating responses to drug abuse. It established the ACMD, a body of independent experts, many of whose recommendations on treatment, rehabilitation, and prevention were reflected in government strategy (Home Office, 1986).

Changing views of drug use and drug problems

Problematic drug use is seen less as the symptom of an illness and more as an example of the wider normal human activity of drug taking. It is more helpful to see it in its widest social and psychological context and to see its effects in many areas of life. Given the diversity of the causes of, and problems arising from, drug use, the range of services must be equally diverse, and able to respond flexibly. The ACMD *Treatment and Rehabilitation* report (1982) adopted a wide definition of problem drug taking: 'any person who experiences social, psychological, physical, or legal problems related to intoxication and/or regular excessive consumption and/or dependence as a consequence of his own use of drugs or other chemical substances (excluding alcohol)'. The consequences of such a wide definition include the need for problem-oriented, rather than disease-oriented treatments, and the involvement of a range of professions. The perspective of the stages of change model (described by Tober in this volume) has led to acceptance of the fluctuating nature of motivation, and the need for readily available, appropriate services capable of intervening in times of crisis.

The development of CDTs

The key impetus to the development of CDTs was the Central Funding Initiative, which established a £17 million pump-priming fund for local projects in England. Many services were set up as a result of this financial initiative, with eighteen projects approximating to the CDT model obtaining £2.545 million, or an average of £141,000 per team spread over three years. The intention was that local Health and Social Services would assume funding thereafter. Two of the teams described below are beneficiaries of the pump-priming monies, while members of the Rochdale CDT are funded by their individual employers on time-limited contracts.

In some health regions, as envisaged by the ACMD in 1982, Regional Drug Problem Teams play an important part in providing a multidisciplinary model for district services, and for setting these up. In the North-West Region, Rochdale can compare its work with nineteen similar teams, and a weekly seminar is held for drug workers in the region. In South-West Thames there are four CDTs, and in Wessex four services on the CDT model.

Current practice in three teams

The descriptions which follow look at three examples of current practice, teams set up in 1985 and 1986 in different parts of England. They focus on the contexts of the teams (in terms of the social setting, the drug 'scene' in the area, and pre-existing and co-existing drug services), the teams and their clients, and the services provided, together with issues of immediate concern. These are snapshots of different services which are still developing, in their second or third year of operation, using opportunities to create better services.

The context of the teams

Rochdale

The Rochdale Health District covers a population of 206,300 people living in the three distinct townships of Rochdale, Heywood, and Middleton, on the northern edge of Greater Manchester, adjoining the Pennines. Textile mills still dominate the towns, and this declining industry remains an important employer, together with engineering works, retailing, and commerce. The overall unemployment rate in the spring of 1988 was 12.7 per cent. The drug 'scene' changed dramatically in the late 1970s and early 1980s when heroin became much more widely used; it is estimated that there are at present some 1,500 opiate users in the district, together with an increasing number of amphetamine users. During 1987 there was a noticeable shift away from smoking heroin towards more injection. Many drug takers are involved in petty crime; the 15 per cent of the probation service clients assessed as having problems with opiates have most frequently been convicted of shoplifting, fraud, burglary, and petty theft. Before the CDT began, in July 1985, the only services available for illicit drug users were non-specialist ones – GPs, general psychiatrists based in a general hospital, and the Sheepgate Community, run by a clergyman.

East Dorset

East Dorset has a population of a half a million, most of whom live in the central conurbation of Bournemouth and Poole, with the remainder in the belt of surrounding countryside and small towns such as Wimborne, Wareham, and Swanage. Although Bournemouth has an 'elderly' image, one in four of the population is aged between 18 and 35. The major industries are tourism (in which there is a great deal of seasonal employment) and light engineering. In the spring of 1988 about 6 per cent of the working population were unemployed. There has been a drug 'scene' with a core of opiate abusers since the 1960s, and current estimates are of the order of one thousand serious drug users. Bournemouth was the first place where the abuse of diconal was recorded and the town in which the first British death from AIDS occurred. Cannabis and amphetamine sulphate are fairly widely used in addition to the opiates, mainly heroin. As well as local people using drugs, there is a steady influx of drug users from elsewhere, many of them heroin users from Merseyside. Before the CDT was formed in 1986 there were four local services for problem drug takers. The Dorset Drug Advisory Service (DDAS) operates from an easily accessible base in the town centre, and is staffed by trained volunteers offering advice, information, and befriending. This has been in existence since the late 1960s, and employs a co-ordinator and a part-time secretary. Meta House is a Christian-based residential rehabilitation centre for female drug takers, with an adjacent house, the Hannah Project, for mothers and children. Meta and Hannah offer an eight-month rehabilitation programme and act as a national resource. There is an out-patient prescribing clinic run on three sessions a week by a consultant psychiatrist with clinical assistant back-up, providing medical assessment and treatment, with access to in-patient beds in an acute ward of the local psychiatric hospital. There is also a strong branch of Narcotics Anonymous which has several meetings a week, including one within the prescribing clinic.

West Surrey and North-East Hampshire

This area is very mixed in character. There are many wealthy, suburban, leafy lanes; but there are also large pockets of social and economic deprivation, and high unemployment. Many people commute to London, and the main local industries are high-tech computer firms; there is also the home of the British Land Army, and other large MOD establishments. The main towns are Aldershot, Camberley, and Farnborough, with many surrounding villages, making a total population of about a quarter of a million. The proportion of young people is high, and new housing is rapidly being built. The unemployment rate in the spring of 1988 was about 3 per cent. The centre of the district is about 35 miles from central London, which is where, according to the police, much of the local street drugs are obtained. Surveys by the CDT have identified 420 illicit drug users in the district; heroin, methadone, amphetamines, and benzodiazepines are widely used, most often, apparently, in the areas of high-density housing and lower incomes on the Hampshire side of the district.

Before the CDT was established most illicit users received help either from London clinics or from the psychiatric hospital in a neighbouring district which offers out-patient prescribing and limited in-patient detoxification. A community physician ran a non-prescribing counselling service for young people, mainly solvent abusers, on one afternoon a week. There were also two small parents' support groups, and a few GPs who were willing to help drug users.

The teams and their clients

Rochdale

The team consists of a social worker, a nurse, a probation officer, a 'Lifeline' field worker, and a voluntary worker, and is supported by a part-time secretary. It is based in a building (originally the lodge) at the entrance to a general hospital which is located at one end of the district. The team functions in a democratic way, without a team leader or manager within it; authority shifts as members defer to discussion and individuals' expertise. Policy and planning is carried out by the Drug Steering Group which meets three times annually, and is chaired by the health authority. The team has had contact with 260 problem drug takers, 90 per cent of them opiate users; during 1987 members came into contact with ninety-four individuals for the first time.

East Dorset

The team consists of a clinical psychologist, a community psychiatric nurse, a social worker, a probation officer, and an occupational therapist. In July 1986 the first three of these were in post; the team was complete in September 1986. They are supported by two part-time secretaries, and share one large office. They see clients in Health Service and Social Services accommodation, which includes a bungalow in hospital grounds on three days a week. The psychologist acts as team leader, co-ordinating the work of the team, although each member is accountable to their line-manager. A code of multidisciplinary teamwork has been accepted by the managers.

Drug takers using the service have typically been in their twenties and early thirties (with a mean age of 28). During the first twelve months of operation 57 per cent of clients had problems with opiates (mainly heroin) and 22 per cent with stimulants (mainly amphetamine sulphate). A large number (57 per cent) took their drugs by injection. Half of the team's contacts took place in clients' homes, half in their own premises. Some in-patient contacts are made in the local psychiatric hospital, some in the regional detoxification unit at

Portsmouth (at which East Dorset fills a higher proportion of regional beds than any other district).

West Surrey and North-East Hampshire

The core team consists of a clinical psychologist, a social worker, a community psychiatric nurse, and an administrator/secretary. The psychologist is the project manager. It is based in offices run jointly by Social and Health Services in a community setting. Clients are seen either in their own homes or in one of three 'drop-in' centres. A grand opening was held in October 1986, with lots of good publicity, and the team has continued to maintain a high public profile through posters and newspaper articles.

During the first 18 months of operation 53 per cent of clients were taking illicit drugs, 33 per cent had problems with benzodiazepines, and 10 per cent abused solvents. Two-thirds of the users of illicit drugs were taking opiates, but only a third of these were taking heroin; methadone was much more common. The illicit users were aged between 16 and 36, with twice as many males as females. The tranquilliser dependent clients were predominantly women, from 35 to 60 years of age; lorazepam was the primary problem drug for 37 per cent of these, and diazepam for another 36 per cent. Most clients refer themselves, although the service may have been recommended to them by GPs, probation officers, or other professionals.

The service

Rochdale

A major task has been enlisting the aid of GPs to provide methadone detoxification programmes for opiate users. One member of the team describes this work:

> We feel like our clients do as we plead and try to persuade their GPs to drop their fears, ignorance, and policy of showing drug users the door and following the shorter guideline of just saying 'No'. Some GPs are very keen and very good, and are probably better able to assess their patients' needs and negotiate an appropriate form of treatment than the team could. GPs who do not 'just say no' risk being swamped by demands from new and temporary patients. By working with the CDT the GP can usually better negotiate treatment programmes which are more likely to be stuck to and lead into a systematic approach to both treatment and counselling.

The team has also led to initiatives for newly-abstinent and recent ex-users. The Rework Project employs eighteen former drug users in the renovation and French polishing of furniture to professional standards. This community programme scheme developed out of the team's concern to tackle the practical needs of people who have recently stopped using, who may be vulnerable, and often have to cope with debts and poverty. They need to do something to fill the gap that abstinence leaves in their lives. Participation in the Rework Project offers a job for a year and, for some, a chance to get a work record to follow a criminal record; this can be a year's intensive support and rehabilitation via work. It employs twenty-eight workers in all, plus five staff. The thirty clients who have been employed have reduced their drug use and their offending; some have gone on to permanent jobs and are doing well.

Another project initiated by the CDT has been sheltered 'drug-free' housing which would enable clients to stay in the area and retain their support in the local community. The idea for this residential project originated with the team; finance was obtained from Urban Aid, and property from a housing association. Turning Point, a voluntary organisation, agreed to undertake the management of the scheme, which is due to open in the spring of 1989.

A third project which the team helped start was FRODA (Friends and Relatives of Drug Abusers), a self-help group which meets on a regular basis to help its members to cope with their burden and occasionally generate action from statutory services.

The CDT helped establish a practical needle-exchange scheme, utilising chemists' shops, and had to consider how to operate a policy of harm reduction in co-ordination with a service aimed at abstention. Even before the ACMD (1988) report on drugs and AIDS was produced, the team reached the conclusion that preventing the spread of HIV must come before any drug-specific goals. This has raised the issue of the attractiveness of the abstinence-oriented service to many users.

East Dorset

Most of the clinical work is done with individuals, although there are groups for opiate users on out-patient detoxification and benzodiazepine withdrawal groups. Before the CDT was set up it had been assumed that its main task would be to provide a treatment and rehabilitation service to drug users who had been detoxified by the prescribing clinic. It became clear that this was unrealistic because so few patients of that clinic completed straightforward detoxification. During the first year of operation clinic patients could freely choose whether or not to use the services of the CDT, and many chose not to. At the end of that year the team opted for closer integration of their work; selected opiate users were offered integrated packages of psychosocial help and a prescription for methadone, the latter being made dependent on the former. This resulted in more group work, which had the unexpected spin-off of attracting a number of amphetamine users who had recently stopped, and were not receiving any medication. It will soon be possible to see whether this approach results in more completed detoxifications and better outcome.

The team has tried several projects which appeared to be promising; some proved successful, some not. One failure was a women's group, for female drug takers, run by two female members of staff in response to the requests of many women clients. Despite arranging crèche facilities and free transport, it was never used by more than three women. One successful project was in helping the formation of a local branch of Families Anonymous, a self-help group for the relatives and close friends of drug users. The team helped by generating appropriate publicity in the media, publicising it to potential members, and helping with accommodation.

In East Dorset injecting drug users are able to buy needles and syringes through retail pharmacies. The CDT co-operates with the local pharmaceutical committee in arranging for pharmacists selling syringes to add to each pack a printed card containing advice about safer sex and safer drug use, and details of local drugs and AIDS agencies. It also arranged a series of two-day intensive skills workshops on AIDS counselling open to members of statutory and non-statutory services. Close links have also been developed with the local AIDS-line and Body Positive Group.

West Surrey and North-East Hampshire

When the CDT was set up as the main drug service in the district, a decision was taken not to include a medical specialist, but instead to provide a helping service that could get away from prescribing and attract drug users for non-medical help. Illicit drug users are offered help on an individual basis, while tranquilliser users are initially offered group counselling and support.

A key-worker system operates with frequent clinical meetings where multidisciplinary discussion of each client enables the team to provide the most suitable service, utilising a wide range of skills and flexible approaches to therapy. The help given to clients by the team varies widely according to whether the client abuses illicit drugs or prescribed tranquillisers. Input assessments show that there has been far more 'behind the scenes' work with the former group, involving advocacy, liaison, and practical forms of interventions, according to their many needs.

The service has, from its very beginning, employed an evaluation system, to justify its existence and to obtain future funding. The evaluations have proved morale-boosting, because they show the service to be relatively effective. Baseline measures of drug use are established for each client at the beginning of treatment, comparing his or her use of each drug during the previous month with that over the previous year. These measures are repeated each month during treatment and then after treatment has ended, and three, six, and twelve months later. Each measurement of drug use is assigned to one of six categories; not known/increased usage/no change/ reduced usage (by less than half the original amount)/greatly reduced usage (by more than half the original amount)/abstinent. The short-term outcome was that 47 per cent of illicit drug users contacting the service had either reduced or stopped their drug use one month after first contact. In the longer term, at the twelve month follow-up, just over half of illicit (mainly opiate) drug users, and two-thirds of tranquilliser users, had reduced their intake or stopped using. Half of the injecting drug users had stopped injecting.

The team has a part-time worker specialising in HIV and AIDS, with particular emphasis on harm reduction. Proposals for a needle-exchange scheme did not win favour with senior Health Service managers and, therefore, following a survey of local pharmacists, the team is looking at the possibility of increasing the availability of injecting equipment through local retail pharmacists.

Another development under serious consideration is the provision of a prescribing service as a means of attracting those users who may not wish to reduce their drug consumption, particularly chaotic young users who are most at risk from infectious diseases. This departure from the original philosophy of a non-medical approach would be justified if it led to greater contact with drug takers who have not used the service. It is felt that a GP employed on a sessional basis would be most compatible with the structure and democratic functioning of the team. The role of this medical practitioner will be to advise clients' GPs on prescribing practice and to take this on in exceptional cases.

Training and consultancy

Rochdale

The team exerts some influence on the delivery of other services through its training functions and by acting as consultants to key workers in contact with clients. It has successfully influenced agencies' policies and informed the practice of workers including housing officers, health visitors, maternity care staff, probation officers, social workers, employment officers, local councillors, neighbourhood workers, as well as relatives and friends of clients. As a result of the work of the team in advising and training maternity care staff, pregnant clients generally receive a more friendly and better standard of health care than they did previously.

East Dorset

The CDT provides training for others, particularly generic professional workers who may come into contact with drug users from time to time. It runs courses every six months on 'Working with drug users' attended by nurses, probation officers, social workers, supervisors of Community Programme (CP) projects, members of voluntary agencies, and others. The success of these courses has been ensured by the involvement of other local drug workers including the DDAS, Meta, Drug Squad, Narcotics Anonymous (NA), the consultant psychiatrist responsible for the prescribing clinic, and Body Positive. Course members are invited to the Drug Interest Group, monthly lunchtime meetings open to all who work with drug problems. This provides continuing education and a regular meeting place, with local and national speakers. During the past twelve months these have included a Home Office Inspector, representatives of local rehabilitation centres, members of the Regional Drug Problem Team, the regional fieldworker from the Standing Committee on Drug Abuse (SCODA), and members of NA. The team has organised training events for its own needs and made them available to drug workers nationally; these have included skills workshops on motivational interviewing, groupwork, and benzodiazepine withdrawal. It has also made two training videos, one on the work of the CDT, the other (with Henck van Bilsen) on motivational interviewing.

West Surrey and North-East Hampshire

Other staff are occasionally attached to the team, either for specific clients or for training placements, including student youth and community workers, nurses, and clinical psychologists. The team has provided courses, workshops, and seminars for statutory agency staff (mainly health professionals, social workers, and probation officers) and volunteers, mostly geared towards training such skills as relapse prevention training and motivational interviewing. The team also organised the Substance Abuse Forum, a monthly seminar with guest speakers, which proved popular.

Evaluating practice

'Pioneering Community Teams must almost inevitably work on a number of fronts. Equally they have to recognise the potential for conflict between their tasks.' Thus commented the Social Services Inspectorate report on drug services in 1985, after examining three new CDTs (Social Services Inspectorate 1985). Where in the three teams described above do we encounter potential or actual conflict?

Management

Of the teams looked at by the Social Services Inspectorate, management structures presented anomalies which are also evident in the three CDTs presented above. Conflict is more likely to arise within multiprofessional teams when the line-managers of team members play a significant part in directing their work. The more that team management is devolved to team members, or to a nominated individual within the team, the more the team can operate as a service delivery unit with scope for experimenting with new forms of service and responding to the needs of clients. During the first two years of each of the CDTs described there was a great deal of experimentation and evolution: there is much value in management arrangements which provide such committed teams with the scope to test out their ideas for service delivery and develop the service accordingly. These management issues for CDTs are not unique and, as Clement's chapter (Chapter 11 in this volume) argues, there is much to learn from the experience of CATs and other multiagency, multiprofessional Community Teams. The management arrangements for the three teams differ considerably: one is a democratic team with joint accountability to a steering group, one has a leader who co-ordinates the service, and the third has a budget-holding project manager. Each arrangement has advantages and disadvantages which have been discussed in detail by Overtreit (1986). The potential for conflict is greater the more informal the relationships between the agencies forming the team: clear formal agreements are helpful in promoting effective teamwork.

Multidisciplinary issues

The arguments for a multiprofessional service are to offer an integrated approach by members of different professions and agencies, each bringing a range of skills. When this works well it can provide a stimulating and creative working environment for its members and break down professional boundaries. Each of the teams described here has had the advantage of promoting multidisciplinary working from the beginning, without the burden of past difficulties. Each has needed to clarify the roles of members and establish procedures for working together which make a team a team and not a collection of individuals. When such teams are working well there tend to be few conflicts about roles or 'demarcation' disputes, but instead a high degree of role blurring. When teams work badly there are disputes about what work is whose. There needs to be agreement within the team about roles, and also agreement with team managers about leadership, but also about roles in teamwork. A social work manager who defines the role of the social worker in a drug team in a very narrow way as only carrying out specific social work tasks limits the scope of agreement within the team. Individual members of the team each come with specific skills and strengths; some of these can be predicted from their profession (are profession-specific) while others are not. Certain skills are developed or extended once in post, again usually regardless of their profession. There needs to be agreement about who does what based on the individuals in post; very few tasks can only be carried out adequately by members of particular professions. It is essential that these roles be agreed, even if informally. Major unresolved disagreements about roles impede the service provided by teams.

Prescribing

The prescription of methadone has been relevant to the treatment of problem opiate takers who comprise the majority of the teams' clients, yet none of the teams contains a medical practitioner who can provide this. Each team has had different access to and relationships with prescribers; in two cases this relationship has had to be re-thought. In East Dorset the ready access of the CDT to a pre-existing prescribing clinic proved to be double-edged because, although the clinic attracted many opiate users, the attraction was often towards the 'script' rather than the help that the CDT was offering. The team decided to move away from its initial separation from the medical service, which had allowed clients the right to choose the drug and reject the team, towards close integration which took away that right from many clients. The team in West Surrey and North-East Hampshire has had to reconsider its initial non-medical stance in order to try and attract more drug users. It and the Rochdale team had to expend much energy in liaising with GPs to gain access to prescriptions for their clients. The comments by the Rochdale team member about trying to get GPs to go beyond 'just saying no' to drug users illustrate the importance of advocacy and the amount of time and effort that can be involved in working with GPs. The more that CDT members become involved in decisions about prescribing, the more potential conflicts can arise for them (involving the issues discussed in Wilks's chapter in this volume). Conflicts are involved between offering a non-medical service for the minority who wish to make use of it and offering access to prescriptions in order to attract (and hopefully influence) a wider range of drug users. To prescribe or not to prescribe is an issue which is still open to some, and the decision taken determines consumers' perceptions of the service provided by the team, as well as the team's relation to other services in the locality.

A service for whom?

To what extent should CDTs attempt to offer a direct service to clients, and to what extent an indirect service, working through other professionals who are in contact with drug users? To what extent should teams restrict their service to users of illicit drugs or open it to problem benzodiazepine users? These issues about goals of services represent further potential conflicts. The first issue, of acting directly or indirectly, has been much more important for CATs than CDTs: the initial model for CATs was as a consultative and training service, with the goal of influencing more generic professionals to work with problem drinkers. In practice CATs, set up with this aim, ended up spending much of their time taking direct referrals, finding the purely consultative role difficult to sustain (as illustrated in Clement's chapter). The three CDTs described have taken direct client work as their major role (two are the only drug service in their district) but have seen training and influencing others as very important. Others, particularly in the north-west of England, have argued that direct client work should be seen as less important. For instance Gillman (1987) puts the point of view that CDTs should encourage others to work with drug users:

> A conference of CDTs, held in January 1986, seemed to establish the principle that 'successful' teams would be those who did not accumulate a high caseload but who ensured that generic services who have problem drug users on their caseload did their best to manage them without referring them to specialist units. This was seen to be especially important if the demystification of drugs and drug users is to be achieved.

The extent to which teams holding this definition of success are able to implement it remains to be determined.

Two of the teams described provide a service for people dependent on tranquillisers, the other (Rochdale) refers such problems to a local Tranx group. Those dependent on tranquillisers differ in many ways from people dependent on illicit drugs, although the latter often also use and abuse minor tranquillisers, as well as alcohol. The suffering produced by withdrawal from tranquillisers is often more intense and drawn out than that from opiates, yet there are few services for those who wish for help with withdrawal. Similar skills are needed to treat problems arising from each category of drug, an overlap often stressed in the training offered to others by drug workers. Teams set up to provide a service to 'problem drug takers' often see tranquilliser problems as within their remit, and often a pleasant change from their other work. The scale of unmet need is so great that, for these problems, the arguments for training and supporting others seem particularly convincing. The argument against working with tranquillisers is that CDTs could easily be swamped by these legal drugs and that, in the light of AIDS, their first priority must be to injecting drug users.

These two areas of conflict concern goals and priorities. Clarifying and agreeing the team's goals, and revising these periodically, is an important process in developing an effective service.

The future of CDTs

In 1988 there were nearly sixty CDTs in England. Their distribution is uneven, some regions have generated more teams, and this does not necessarily reflect the distribution of drug problems. The adage applied to drug squads is also true of drug services: 'If you haven't got one, you haven't got a drug problem'. To some extent the development of CDTs has occurred where there were few or no voluntary agencies in existence, and a gap to be filled.

The report of the ACMD working party on drugs and AIDS, published in the spring of 1988, argues that community services should be substantially developed and expanded. Their objectives should be to make contact with drug users for the purpose of harm minimisation, and to reduce the risk of the spread of HIV infection. The epidemiology of AIDS will continue to influence the perceived need for CDTs. While injecting drug users are a relatively high-risk group, it is seen as reasonable to invest in prevention in this group. If the disease becomes widespread in the non-drug-using population, however, or if it should recede entirely, priorities may change. The future of many CDTs is limited by the three years of pump-priming funding. In many cases decisions about future funding by Health and Social Services will depend on evaluations of their effectiveness. Popular criteria such as the number of abstinent former drug users are probably too simple. Is the effectiveness of GPs judged by the number of perfectly healthy people on their lists? Other indicators of the usefulness of CDTs might include the number of community-based detoxifications completed, reduction in drug use, stabilisation, a step from injection to oral use, the client's own assessment of his or her progress towards selected goals, and the use made of the CDT by other agencies; all need to be taken into consideration. Three years is a relatively short time in a drug-using career, not only for illicit drug users, who appear to spend a median number of ten years using drugs. Tranquilliser dependency can also last for many years – ten is not uncommon – and withdrawal programmes lasting longer than twelve months are often undertaken. Building a drug-free life is a long-term task; so is developing effective services able to respond flexibly to the changing patterns of drug use and needs of drug users.

References

Advisory Council on the Misuse of Drugs (1982) *Treatment and Rehabilitation*, London: HMSO.

Advisory Council on the Misuse of Drugs (1988) *AIDS and Drug Misuse, Part 1*, London: HMSO.

DHSS (1984) *Guidelines of good clinical practice in the treatment of drug misusers*, London: HMSO.

Gillman, M. (1987) 'Community Drug Teams', *Mersey Drug Journal*, 1: 11–12.

Home Office (1986) *Tackling drug misuse: A summary of the government's strategy*, 2nd edn, London: HMSO.

Overtreit, J. (1986) *Organisation of multidisciplinary community teams*, Brunel Institute of Organisational Studies (BIOSS), Brunel University.

Social Services Inspectorate (1985) 'Project on drug misuse', unpublished report.

Chapter Eleven

The Community Drug Team: lessons from alcohol and handicap services

Sue Clement

Introduction

Over the last decade the formation of specialist community teams has been an increasing trend in the over-all picture of service provision for a number of client groups. Community Alcohol Teams (CATs) and Community Mental Handicap Teams (CMHTs) are the most widely-established examples of this trend, with Community Drug Teams (CDTs) and Community Elderly Teams (CETs) being a more recent phenomenon. Whilst there is a growing literature relating to CMHTs and CATs, little has been written about Community Drug Teams. Most of the published work relates to *process* (that is, difficulties in setting up and running teams) rather than to *outcome* issues. Those studies which have attempted to evaluate outcome have tended to focus on the impact of community teams on primary workers rather than on evaluating the extent to which this form of service delivery is beneficial to clients. Where benefits to clients are asserted these tend to be couched in terms of improved access to less stigmatising services rather than in terms of improved outcome, an area which remains to be vigorously evaluated.

The development of specialist community teams is occurring against a background of increasing concern about the entire concept of community care which has been criticised by both the Commons Social Services Committee in 1985[1] and the Audit Commission in 1986.[2] Many of the problems identified by the Audit Commission in the general organisation of community care are also referred to in the community team literature. They concern fundamental questions about the way in which services are organised and managed. Because of the multidisciplinary nature of the majority of specialist community teams they provide a series of case studies which enable some of the difficulties resulting from attempts at interagency co-operation and management to be examined. They also provide an insight into some of the difficulties and strengths of multidisciplinary team-working at the field-work level. The striking similarities between issues raised in both the CAT and CMHT literature suggest that any specialist community team can learn from the lessons of others, regardless of the nature of the client population they purport to serve. The concern with process rather than outcome variables in the literature illustrates that many of these common concerns relate to how one sets up and introduces a novel form of service delivery within an already established structure, a question of immediate relevance to CDTs.

The policy framework

The role of CATs was first outlined in the series of reports made to DHSS by the Maudsley Alcohol Pilot Project (MAPP). An examination of these reports, however, finds a progressive narrowing of the role advocated for CATs. The 1975 report argued that the CAT should take over-all responsibility for the initiation and co-ordination of the model service described[3] which 'mobilized and integrated the potential skills of a variety of services, generic and specialist, at both primary and secondary levels'. The CAT was also expected to play a role in service development (this model of CATs closely paralleled the later proposals for Regional Drug Problem Teams put forward by the Advisory Council on the Misuse of Drugs in 1982)[4] and those put forward by the National Development Team in the late 1970s regarding Community Mental Handicap Teams,[5] although there was a greater emphasis in both the latter on teams providing direct services to clients. By 1978, however, there was little mention of the role of the CAT in either service development or co-ordination.[6] What was emphasised was a much more specific brief, to facilitate the involvement of primary care workers with problem drinkers through the provision of training and role support, much closer in effect to the role advocated by the Advisory Council on the Misuse of Drugs for the District Drug Problem Team. Whilst the Advisory Committee on Alcoholism (ACA) in their 1978 report[7] recognised the need for better co-ordinated services, they did not see the CAT as taking on this role (indeed the phrase, Community Alcohol Team, does not appear, although references are made to a need to establish 'local teams'). The ACA felt that co-ordination was best achieved by a specialist subgroup appointed by the Joint Care Planning Team which should be responsible for finding 'ways for both formal links between the agencies to be made and for their individual members to work together'. The role of the 'local team', comprising as a minimum a psychiatrist – perhaps part-time – , nurse, social worker, and voluntary counsellor, all with specialist skills, remained ill-defined from the role outlined in general for secondary level specialist services. Central policy guidelines then provided little specific guidance to service planners on what CATs were meant to do whilst the work of the MAPP appeared to offer contradictory messages.

Although the Advisory Council on the Misuse of Drugs made much clearer recommendations regarding the role of community teams than the earlier report by the Advisory Committee on Alcoholism, both documents failed to specify in any great detail the underlying principles they felt should guide service development. Although such principles as meeting a range of client need and accessibility of services were often implicit in what was said, neither report put forward the kind of coherent and comprehensive statement of principles which is available within policy documents relating to services for the mentally handicapped. An early example of such a statement are the fifteen general principles covering a wide range of important issues relating to service planning and provision outlined in the 1971 White Paper, *Better Services for the Mentally Handicapped*.[8] Subsequent reports have also addressed this issue and in 1980 the National Development Group[9] produced a checklist of the questions and issues that need to be addressed by agencies and individuals concerned with developing, improving, or evaluating services for mentally-handicapped people. In contrast, there are few structured guidelines available to people concerned with developing and running substance misuse services. The lack of such principles makes it difficult to evaluate the extent to which services are meeting their over-all aims. A recent attempt to formulate certain key principles which should underlie a comprehensive approach to tackling alcohol problems[10] at a local level came up with the following:

> Prevention is better than cure – if this is not possible early intervention is preferable to trying to deal with problems once they have become more severe.
>
> Services should be flexible – people develop alcohol problems for many different reasons and therefore their needs cannot be met in a uniform way. Services should offer a variety of responses to their clients.
>
> Clients should have some choice – there should be enough services available to enable clients to choose between at least two different types of help.

> Services should respect clients' rights – issues such as confidentiality, the right to be heard properly, adequate privacy in residential settings, should all be fully taken account of.
>
> Labelling and stigmatising should be avoided – every attempt should be made to avoid the dangers of increasing people's problems by labelling them in a certain way and seeing them as quite different to the rest of society.
>
> Services should start with people's needs and be planned on that basis.
>
> Monitoring and evaluations should form a part of the service – even if this is only done at a very basic level.
>
> (Alcohol Services Information Pack. Alcohol Concern 1987)

Such a list of principles, however, has not been made explicit in the policy statements by central government relating to either alcohol or other drug services, as Strang (1985) noted when he commented:

> The Treatment and Rehabilitation Report of the Advisory Council on the Misuse of Drugs recommended adaption of a problem-orientated approach, but many clinicians feel that too little guidance has been given on how such an approach should be used in practice.[11]

The absence of clearly specified principles underlying service development has given service planners little to fall back upon when the service structures recommended have not proved practical to implement at the local level.

Local adaptation

The policy documents advocating the setting up of specialist multidisciplinary teams, whether they are concerned with mentally-handicapped people, alcohol, or other drug misusers, all made recommendations regarding catchment area and staffing. In practice, the teams which have been set up have been found to vary so much in size, disciplinary mix, and population served, that it is difficult to know what is actually meant by the terms CMHT, CAT, or CDT.

Some 'teams' may have only one member, typically a Community Psychiatric Nurse (CPN), whilst others may have upward of twelve members (some giving sessional input, others full-time). Some may be a part of a comprehensive network of local services whilst others may be expected to provide district-wide services in isolation. Few of the teams which have been set up appear to have been given operational policy statements to guide the direction of the work of members. In a recent survey it was found that about three-quarters of CMHTs operating in one Regional Health Authority (RHA) had no operational policy statement.[12] Of the twenty CDTs in another RHA, only a couple were believed to have such operational policies.[13] It is not unusual then for teams not only to be expected to provide a service but also to be expected to work out what it is they should be doing at the same time, with little or no guidance from either local planners, managers, or central government.

A recent survey of CATs which sent a representative to a national CAT conference in 1986 found that, out of the fourteen teams represented, six felt that their primary aim when first set up was to provide a direct service to problem drinkers, five to support primary workers in managing drinkers themselves, and three felt both these aims were equally important.[14] When examining the types of activity in which teams were actually *currently* involved, it was found that all the teams were attempting to pursue both these aims – and often others in addition (see Table 11.1).

Table 11.1 Activities of CATs identified in 1986 survey

Activity	*No. of teams (n = 13)*
Direct client services	13
Support of primary workers	13
Education of primary workers	12
Education of general public	6
Promoting alcohol policies at work	2

Source: T. Stockwell and S. Clement (1986) *Community Alcohol Teams, A Review and Appraisal*, Report to DHSS.

Service development did not appear to be a main priority for any of the teams, although some services such as NORCAS (Norwich CAT), with a county-wide brief, have been successful in developing sister services in a number of other locations. Although the extent and nature of all these activities varied from team to team, what is important to note is the degree of consensus which has emerged about what the role of CATs entails, an issue which was much in question at the first national CAT conference in 1983. A couple of points need to be made, however, in relation to the previous comments regarding operational brief. The survey did not ask to what extent either the initial or subsequently developed aims of the teams were formally recognised in operational policy statements, or to what extent they had been negotiated with management. There is no indication of to what extent teams developed their service goals in a relatively autonomous way or to what extent they reflect clear decisions about changes in goals as opposed to a more general policy of reacting to demands made upon them. Second, there was no indication of how service goals were being prioritised. The emergence of a degree of consensus about broad goals then is not particularly helpful to newly-developing teams, although it remains an interesting finding in itself. However, a number of factors do appear to be relevant in influencing the structure and aims of community teams:

1. Amount and nature of existing service provision

Teams such as Salford CAT initially focused on providing a support service to primary workers rather than seeing clients because other agencies locally were perceived as offering adequate client-orientated services. In contrast, Exeter CAT, formed in 1981, following the closure of the local Alcohol Treatment Unit (ATU), focused on providing a direct client service from a community base.

2. Available resources

The number of full-time team members and the extent to which sessional workers are seconded will be dependent on available funding.

3. Locally identified need both of clients and agencies

What are the gaps in existing service provision and what client needs are currently unmet? Who are the 'clients'? Some CDTs, for example, have become orientated towards providing services for tranx users because there are apparently few illicit drug users in their district.

4. Priority attached to multidisciplinary team development

This will reflect the quality of the relationship between health and local authorities and voluntary organisations, and also the extent to which different groups of workers are perceived as having something valuable to offer to any given team.

5. Philosophy and professional background of service innovators

Given the lack of guidelines available to aid service planners, teams often reflect much of the philosophy of those individuals who have been the prime movers behind their development.

The way these factors have interacted in different localities has resulted in the wide variety of form of service delivery grouped under the heading 'community teams'.

Service goals

A number of tasks can be identified which community teams hold in common whether their clients are the mentally handicapped, drug or alcohol misusers. Not every team would necessarily see every task identified as part of their role, and the emphasis laid on particular tasks will vary from team to team and sometimes within a team itself. It has already been noted that as teams develop the nature of their roles may also change.

The tasks identified include:

(a) Direct work with clients.
(b) Provision of advice, support, and training to others involved with the client.
(c) Service co-ordination or liaison.
(d) Service development.

An additional goal of teams should include some monitoring and evaluation of activities undertaken in the above categories.

Direct work with clients

The Advisory Committee on Alcoholism (1978) saw the impracticality of trying to offer a specialist service to everyone with alcohol-related problems; the numbers would be too large for any specialist service to handle, nor would it always be appropriate. They felt that the majority of people experiencing alcohol-related problems could, when necessary, be offered help at the primary care level with only a small proportion needing to be referred on to secondary level agencies such as the CAT. In practice, however, nearly all CATs have found themselves dealing directly with fairly substantial numbers of clients, as have many CDTs, despite the recommendation of the Advisory Council on the Misuse of Drugs (1982) which had envisaged a more consultative/educational role for them. For some CATs this was a conscious decision, based on local needs in the absence of any other alcohol services. For other teams it occurred almost despite their original intentions. Similar pressures to engage in casework which was not initially envisaged were reported by Wistow and Wray (1986) in their evaluation of the Nottinghamshire CMHTs.[15] They commented on the external pressures on teams from other professionals and clients, and on the internal pressures generated by the interests, commitment, and career development needs of the team members themselves. External pressures from other professionals tend to vary with the degree of organisational closeness between team members and others within their professional group. Team members with the same line-managers as non-specialist members of their own profession seemed to come under the most pressure to engage in direct client work, either from the managers themselves or from their non-specialist colleagues for whom they were easily approachable. Such pressure was found to be particularly difficult to resist when team members felt that the client would receive a greater degree of help from them than could be provided by stretched and less experienced generic workers. When the majority of team members come from case-work oriented backgrounds this kind of argument is particularly seductive, because not only is seeing clients what workers have been trained to do, but taking on the client also provides an opportunity for the team to 'establish credibility' at the field-work level.

'Establishing credibility' or 'building bridges' (between the team and other workers) is anecdotally reported to be behind many of the decisions taken by teams to take on direct client work when it has not been an initial aim of the service. There is no evidence that any community team has been successful in providing a well-utilised consultancy service to primary care workers unless they have also engaged in case-work with clients. Nevertheless, there are dangers for teams taking on direct work with clients, if they also have other priority aims, unless they have some mechanism for controlling the amount of work taken on. Because of the pressures, both internal and external, to work directly on a one-to-one basis with clients, teams can find themselves with little time to engage in other forms of activities unless clearly defined boundaries are agreed upon. Supportive and informed management should have an important role in helping teams maintain agreed boundaries, as it can often be difficult for team members, when faced with immediate client need, to step back and remember the service's wider goals. Another strategy used by many existing teams is to allocate responsibility for non-clinical roles, such as training of primary care workers, to particular team members who carry reduced case-loads as a result.

Provision of advice, support, and training to others

The literature which deals with the involvement of generic primary care workers with the problem drug taker evokes a sense of *déjà-vu* for those familiar with the background to Community Alcohol Teams. The same problems (lack of priority given to the client group, inadequate training and resources, inexperience and lack of support) are invoked to explain lack of worker involvement, and the same solutions (channelling training, support, and advice through multidisciplinary community teams) are proposed. Regardless of client group, all the literature reiterates the need for better basic training in its own particular area of interest, more in-service training, and the need for a higher priority to be given to whatever client group it is referring to. The primary care worker emerges as a scarce resource, upon which conflicting demands are placed by different specialists for a larger slice of the cake. It is not surprising that many primary care agencies have responded less than enthusiastically to the demands of yet one more service to give their client group a higher priority and that the reactions to consultancy services designed to 'improve' individual worker's responses have initially been ones of suspicion.[16]

Despite this there is some evidence from the CAT research that Community Alcohol Teams have achieved some success in changing the negative attitudes of primary workers to working with clients with alcohol problems. Both the Liverpool[17] and Salford[18] evaluations found that primary workers (excluding GPs) identified greater numbers of problem drinkers on their case-loads after the CATs came into operation (an increase of 2.9 per cent in the case of Liverpool and 4.8 per cent in the case of Salford). There is some evidence from the Salford study that GPs were also identifying more problem drinkers. These changes were found to be related, not to an increased awareness of the indicators of problem drinking, but to an increased likelihood that workers would discuss drinking with clients at an earlier stage of their involvement with them.[19] Salford primary workers when interviewed showed a reasonable awareness of the indicators of a drinking problem before being given any training. What was lacking was confidence that they had anything to offer problem drinkers (low therapeutic commitment). As they grew in confidence they became more willing to raise the subject of drinking with clients. As a consequence, the number of clients with drinking problems that workers were aware of on their case-loads increased. Two factors appeared to be responsible for the gain in confidence by the primary workers – their perception that they would be supported by the CAT in their work with the drinker (CAT 'support' could range from one-off case discussion to taking the client on for treatment), and the training in working with drinkers provided by the team (see Figure 11.1).

Whereas workers who were offered clinical support and advice but no training showed no further gains in therapeutic commitment after the first year of the CAT's operation, workers offered training in addition to the support service continued to make further gains, and there is some suggestion that these workers began to deal with a growing number of problem drinkers themselves without having

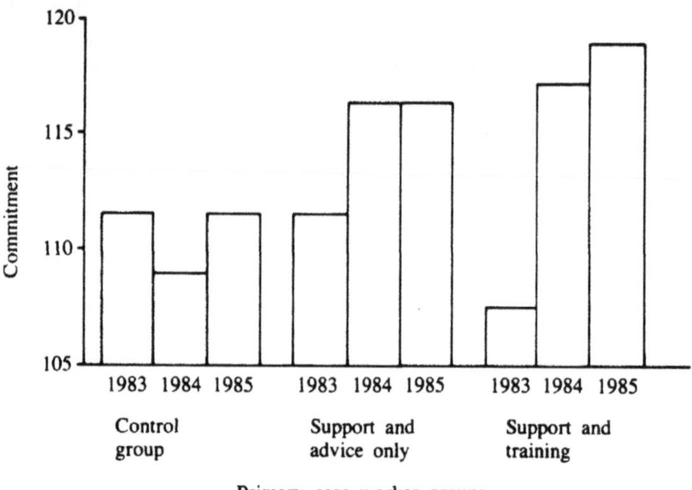

Figure 11.1 Changes in therapeutic commitment found among primary workers in Salford after the CAT's inception in 1983

Source: T. Stockwell and S. Clement (1986) *Community Alcohol Teams. A Review and Appraisal*, Report to DHSS.

recourse to the CAT. The training offered to the primary workers utilised members of the local CAT as teachers, rather than outside experts, and this proved helpful both in terms of building up the relationship between CAT and workers, and in making the training relevant and responsive to the needs of most workers. The training was multidisciplinary in nature and consisted of one-day courses which were repeated, so that every primary worker had a chance to attend without having to shut down offices for the day. The fact that workers who were offered training continued to increase in therapeutic commitment throughout the evaluation period, whereas other workers who were offered only clinical support service did not, shows the importance of offering formal training input to the success of a consultancy type approach. The fact that managers were willing to release staff for training also showed the staff that working with drinkers was considered of some relevance to their main job.

One group of primary workers whom all CATs have experienced difficulty in attracting into training have been GPs. Ineichen and Russell (1980) have reported similar problems. They found a generally negative response by GPs to the offer of more training in mental handicap, although few of their sample had received any.[20]

Table 11.2 Mean number of primary worker referrals per year to CATs

Profession	*Exeter*	*Medway*	*Norwich*	*Liverpool*	*Salford*
Community nursing	6	6	0	5	42.5
GP	44.5	13	61	11	82.5
Probation	14.5	17	17	15	38.5
Social work	7.5	14	17	19	17.5
Total	72.5	49*	95	50	181.0

* Figures rounded to nearest whole number hence discrepant total.

Source: T. Stockwell and S. Clement (1986) *Community Alcohol Teams. A Review and Appraisal*, Report to DHSS.

They suggested that an alternative way of increasing GPs' effectiveness would be to channel appropriate information on handicap and facilities available in their locality to them in written form, a tactic also used by some CATs, although to date there is no evidence that such strategies are effective.

Although GPs have not responded well to training initiatives, they have tended to refer more clients to the CATs so far evaluated than other groups of primary workers (see Table 11.2). In the case of Liverpool and Salford this may reflect the different service offered to GPs who could refer clients to CAT in a traditional manner, without the long degree of continued involvement which was expected from other workers. For other CATs, however, the same service was on offer to all, and the most parsimonious explanation is simply that there are more GPs than other primary workers. Individually, the Salford data showed that each GP made on average 1.6 referrals to the project over two years as compared to 3.9 by probation officers, 5.7 by CPNs and 0.6 by social workers. GPs as a group, however, made 43 per cent of all referrals to the project. The evaluation suggested that GPs referring to the CAT became more likely to run routine blood tests on patients they felt had drinking problems, and less likely to prescribe psychotropic medication unless detoxification were required.[21] There is some evidence then that the practice of GPs can be changed through the provision of community-based support services, even in the absence of formal training input.

Service co-ordination

Although the need for better co-ordination between service sectors has been recognised within the alcohol field, the CAT has not been seen as the vehicle for achieving this. In contrast, CMHTs were specifically set up with a brief to co-ordinate service delivery. In practice, however, CATs have become involved in service co-ordination, particularly at the field-work level, although little to date has been written about this aspect of their role. Brown (1986) has identified three different levels at which service co-ordination is required: co-ordination to surmount service duplication, co-ordination to fill service gaps, and co-ordination to resolve value conflicts.[22] The Individual Programme Plan (IPP) system, the central element in providing a co-ordinated response to the needs of mentally-handicapped people, appears to meet the needs of service co-ordination at all three levels.[23] The basic content of an IPP comprises three elements: preparation, the IPP meeting and follow-up, and review. Each client is allocated a key worker who carries out an initial assessment and then organises a meeting at which workers involved with the client identify what they can and cannot provide in terms of meeting the client's identified needs. The clients themselves are involved in the meeting, which results in a written plan setting out (a) how the identified needs are to be met, (b) who is responsible for doing what, (c) specifies a review date, and (d) identifies what cannot be provided, and passes this information on to service planners. Problems in implementing this system have been discussed elsewhere.[24] It has, however, been noted that these difficulties are minimised when participation in the system has been agreed by all the agencies involved as occurred in Clwyd in regards to the All Wales Strategy (a policy initiative backed up by considerable financial resources seeking to provide better services for mentally-handicapped people).[25] It could be argued in the context of alcohol and other drug services that an IPP system would be easier to sell to agencies than the consultancy type service previously referred to because one of its specific functions is to identify what workers are unable to offer to clients, whereas a consultancy service implicitly supposes that the primary worker has an obligation to remain involved with the client. It addresses the realities of what resources actually are available at the primary care level, and helps identify what tasks generic workers can and cannot take on in a structured fashion. If the system is backed up by a policy document which has been accepted by all the relevant agencies, the likelihood of generic workers participating in the process would be increased.

One of the problems in implementing this kind of approach for any community team, however, is that they are more likely to be in a position where they are expected to *liaise* rather than *co-ordinate*. Brown (1986) argues that a team's ability or inability to co-ordinate services will be reflected in the number of service resources which the team itself controls.[26] Where teams have limited control over resources, their function becomes one of liaison rather than co-ordination because they become involved in mediating between clients and services rather than directing clients to services. They have no control over the availability and quality of other services in such circumstances. Malcolm Payne (1986) places this discussion in its organisational context:[27]

> Various structures for carrying out net-working between organisations can exist: there is a hierarchy, each level being of greater complexity. At the lowest level is *communication*, where the organisations merely keep each other informed. Then at the *co-operation* stage they are prepared to act to help or support one another. This achieved, they are often prepared to move to *co-ordination* where they agree to change their practice activities or boundaries to rationalise their work. Sometimes, later, they are prepared to move on to *federation*, where they keep some independence but manage some activities jointly.

In Payne's terminology then, CMHTs represent the 'federation' stage of networking in so far as they are jointly managed by the different agencies employing CMHT members. However, the over-all service system within which many CMHTs operate is still at the stage of 'co-operation', little thought having been given to the mechanisms whereby the CMHT can facilitate the changes necessary to rationalise work in the over-all system. This mismatch between stages means that the community team is in no position to co-ordinate services, and has to rely on the goodwill of other components of the over-all service in order to carry out a liaison brief. In theory the CMHT promotes the over-all goal of service co-ordination through feeding information to the Joint Care Planning Team. In practice:

> the suspicion remains that rather than creating a 'new order' of local partnerships between service agencies, teams may be caught in the tensions and misunderstandings which produced the fragmented and un-co-ordinated services of the past.[28]

The problems associated with joint planning between local authorities and health authorities have been well documented elsewhere.[29,30,31,32] Of particular relevance to alcohol and other drug services, however, are the findings of a recent survey that whereas 87 per cent of district health authorities had joint planning teams for mental handicap services, only 16 per cent had planning teams concerned with drug and/or alcohol services.[33] The structure within which Community Drug and Alcohol Teams work therefore needs to be considered when looking at the extent to which it is possible for them to operationalise a service co-ordination brief.

Service development

Whereas for CATs the central issue has always been how to strike a balance between service delivery and providing advice, support and training to primary workers, the question of whether service delivery or service development functions should predominate has been the crucial issue for CMHTs. To some extent the distinction is an artificial one as CMHTs, taking their brief from the National Development Group recommendations, have seen *facilitating joint working* between professionals in the actual delivery of services, a task also attempted by some CATs, albeit in a less structured way. The low key nature of much of this work, however, reflects the absence of clear operational guidelines and a facilitative organisational structure.[34] *The development of service infrastructure* has been much less commonly found to be an initial goal of community teams, with the exception of the CMHTs set up in Nottinghamshire.[35] The Notts. experience showed that the team's capacity for further developmental work weakened quickly under the demand to support the newly-developed services, and that the development of a service infrastructure could only be sustained:

(a) by providing CMHTs with staff whose primary task was to support developments;
(b) by transferring the support function to other bodies such as area social work teams, housing agencies, voluntary organisations, and health service.

Wistow and Wray have commented on the implications of these strategies for the extent to which management of services should be decentralised, as well as on the capacity of CMHTs to manage support staff without their developmental role once again becoming silted up.

It has been argued that a third aspect of the developmental role of community teams should be the *mobilisation of informal care*, along the lines suggested by the Barclay Report (1982) which was concerned with the role of Social Services Departments.[36] Allen (1983) has argued that the 'informal network of carers' referred to in the Report is a largely illusory concept because, in reality, most informal care is provided by close family members, principally mothers and daughters, rather than being spread through a network of carers in the 'community'.[37] Two strategies therefore need to be concentrated on:

1. The provision of support for carers through the organising of services such as day centres, sitting services, etc. – that give some respite and freedom from the demands of caring.
2. The establishment and encouragement of self-help groups for those involved in caring who are in similar circumstances and who share similar problems.

Little has been written in the CAT literature about either the development of service infrastructure or the establishment of mutual self-help groups, although there is a wealth of literature which considers the role of Alcoholics Anonymous and Al-Anon which is of relevance here.[38] As with service co-ordination, however, service development is not a task which the community team can undertake in isolation. The support received from service managers and planners is crucial in determining the extent to which such a role can be operationalised.

Team-work issues

It has already been observed that neither CATs, CMHTs, nor CDTs can be distinguished by a single organisational form. Teams differ in size, in professional mix, and in terms of whether they employ full-time staff, receive sessional input, or combine a mixture of both. Equally there are differences between teams in management structure and team accountability. There are, however, some needs which are common to all teams. Because in many areas where community teams have been set up they represent an innovative form of service delivery, there has been a tendency for these needs to remain unmet until problems arise for the team because planners have been unaware of the importance of setting initial boundaries, objectives, and priorities. Very often the line-managers of team members are not involved in the planning groups which propose teams, and may be unclear as to their relationship with the team.[39]

Overtreit (1986) identified a number of typical problems which community team members often report:[40]

(a) difficulty exerting anything more than peer-group pressure over team members who do not follow team policies;
(b) poor case co-ordination within the team and poor liaison with others involved in a case;
(c) difficulty formulating, agreeing, and following priorities between different types of work (for example, proportion of time on direct case work);
(d) uneven and unfair work distribution between team members;

(e) long-term cases not properly reviewed or closed;
(f) high case-loads preventing the team developing into other areas of work;
(g) uncertainty about the role of the team in relation to general services, and about how the team fits into the over-all service and strategy.

Most of these difficulties reflect the lack of a clearly-defined and agreed management structure, both at the team level and in terms of the over-all service delivery system. Although it is recognised that some team members may see disadvantages in a clearly-defined structure, without it the advantages of team-work to clients can be seen to be minimised whilst staff are left unsupported and uncertain about their roles. Three main areas need to be addressed in whatever structure is agreed: case co-ordination, work-load management, and staff management. To define these arrangements it is necessary to be clear about the work to be done and how the work responsibilities are divided between (a) a 'key worker', (b) a team leader, (c) the team meeting, or the team as a corporate group, and (d) professional superiors outside the team. Overtreit (1986) argues that the authority of each group should stem from the work each has to do, and should be clearly specified and agreed by all involved. Authority can range from authority to request a piece of work or information from another person right through to authority to overrule or make a variety of key decisions.

In addition to creating a management structure which facilitates productive work, attention also needs to be given to what is called 'multidisciplinary team building'. In writing about mental-handicap teams, Ash and Woods comment:

> Just as it is unrealistic to expect a camel (which has been described as a horse designed by a committee) to win the Grand National at the first attempt, so perhaps it is unrealistic to assemble a collection of different disciplines and to expect them to function immediately as an efficient team.[41]

Team building calls on members to develop, not only their own professional skills, but also an understanding of the role of other disciplines and the over-all role, tasks, and function of the team. Beyond that the team needs to develop the shared values, knowledge, and skills necessary for effective multidisciplinary team-work. This does not happen automatically, and traditional professional training leaves team members ill-equipped to face this challenge. It is an area which all too frequently is ignored in the training (if any) which is offered to teams.

Conclusion

Given the difficulties which have faced multidisciplinary community teams, it seems almost a miracle that any have survived. The central issue is how these teams can be integrated into the existing service structure in such a way as to not only enhance the over-all pattern of service provision, but also to facilitate and support the work done by the team. If this is going to happen we need to be much clearer about what the needs of our client group are, and how we propose to meet them. The fact that so many teams have survived is a tribute to the adaptability and commitment of their individual members. In order to sustain their commitment the teams themselves need to receive the support and commitment of others. If we cannot learn this lesson from existing teams the future of community services looks bleak.

Notes

1. House of Commons Second Report from the Social Services Committee (1985) *Community Care with Special Reference to Adult Mentally Ill and Mentally Handicapped People*, London: HMSO.
2. Audit Commission for Local Authorities in England and Wales (1986) *Making a Reality of Community Care*, London: HMSO.
3. Maudsley Alcohol Pilot Project (1975) *Designing a Comprehensive Community Response to Problems of Alcohol Abuse*, Report to DHSS.
4. Advisory Council on the Misuse of Drugs (1982) *Treatment and Rehabilitation*, London, HMSO.
5. Development Team for the Mentally Handicapped (1978) *First Report 1976–1977*, London: HMSO.
6. Shaw, S., Cartwright, A., Spratley, T., and Harwin, J. (1978) *Responding to Drinking Problems*, London: Croom Helm.
7. Advisory Committee on Alcoholism (1978) *The Pattern and Range of Services for Problem Drinkers*, London: DHSS and Welsh Office.
8. Department of Health and Social Security (1971) *Better Services for the Mentally Handicapped*, Cmnd 7468, London: HMSO.
9. National Development Group for the Mentally Handicapped (1980) *Improving the Quality of Services for Mentally Handicapped People. A Checklist of Standards*, London: DHSS.
10. Alcohol Concern (1987) *Alcohol Services Information Pack*.
11. Strang, J. (1985) 'Breaking out of Procrustes Bed – services for problem drug takers', *Bulletin of the Royal College of Psychiatrists*, 9.
12. Brown, S. (1987) *Team Profiles. Towards a Register of Community Mental Handicap Teams*, Report to DHSS.
13. Donmall, M. (1987), personal communication.

14. Stockwell, T. and Clement, S. (1986) *Community Alcohol Teams. A Review and Appraisal*, Report to DHSS.
15. Wistow, G. and Wray, K. (1986) 'CMHT's service delivery and service development: the Nottinghamshire approach', in Grant, G., Humphreys, S., and Magrath, M. (eds) *Community Mental Handicap Teams. Theory and Practice*, British Institute of Mental Handicap Conference Services.
16. Clement, S. (1987) The Salford experiment', in Stockwell, T. and Clement, S. (eds) *Helping the Problem Drinker, New Initiatives in Community Care*, London: Croom Helm.
17. O'Hara, P. (1986) *The Liverpool Alcohol Community Team*, Report to DHSS.
18. Clement, S. (1987) *An Evaluation of the Salford Community Alcohol Team*, Report to Salford Health Authority and DHSS.
19. Ibid.
20. Ineichen, B. and Russell, J.A.O. (1980) *Mental Handicap and Community Care – the View Point of the General Practitioner*, Mental Handicap Studies, Research Report no. 4, University of Bristol, Development of Mental Health.
21. Clement, S. (see note 18).
22. Brown, S. (1986) *Community Mental Handicap Teams. Organisation, Operation and Outcomes*, Interim Report to DHSS.
23. Humphreys, S. (1986) 'Individual planning in NIMROD', in *Community Mental Handicap Teams. Theory and Practice*, op. cit. (see note 15).
24. Berry, I. (1986) 'Individual programme planning and the All Wales Strategy', in *Community Mental Handicap Teams. Theory and Practice*, op. cit. (see note 15).
25. Ibid.
26. Brown, S. (1986) op. cit.
27. Payne, M. (1986) 'Community connections through voluntary organisations. Problems and issues', in *Community Mental Handicap Teams. Theory and Practice*, op. cit. (see note 15).
28. Brown, S. (1986) op. cit.
29. DHSS (1985) *Progress in Partnership.*
30. Harding, T. (1986) *A Stake in Planning, Joint Planning and the Voluntary Sector*, London: National Council of Voluntary Organisations (NCVO).
31. Booth, T.A. (1981) 'Collaboration between the Health and Social Services. A case study of joint care planning', *Policy and Politics*, 9 (1): 23–49.
32. Baldwin, S. (1987) 'New wine in old bottles', in *Helping the Problem Drinker, New Initiatives in Community Care*, op. cit. (see note 16).
33. Harding, T., op. cit.
34. Brown, S. (1987) *Case Management Practice. An Examination of Casework in CMHTs*, Interim Report to DHSS.
35. Wistow, G. and Wray, K. op. cit.

36. Barclay Report (1982) *Social Workers: Their Role and Tasks*, London: Bedford Square Press.
37. Allen, G. (1983) 'Informal networks of care: issues raised by Barclay', *Journal of Social Work*, 13: 417, 433.
38. Robinson, D. (1979) *Talking out of Alcoholism: The Self Help Process*, London: Croom Helm.
39. Overtreit, J. (1986) *Organisation of Multi-disciplinary Community Teams*, BIOSS Working Paper, Brunel University.
40. Ibid.
41. Ash, A. and Woods, P.A. (1986) 'Courses for horses. Foundation course for CMHT members', in *Community Mental Handicap Teams: Theory and Practice*, op. cit. (see note 15).

Name index

Subject index

Milton Keynes UK
Ingram Content Group UK Ltd.
UKHW040013071024
449327UK00011B/203